The Essentials of Anatomy, Sanitary Science and Embalming

A Series

By Asa Johnson Dodge

For twelve years Lecturer and Demonstrator of the Massachusetts College of Embalming.

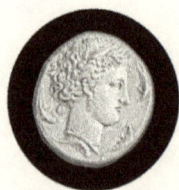

PANTIANOS
CLASSICS

Published by Pantianos Classics

ISBN-13: 978-1-78987-499-0

First published in 1906

Contents

Disclaimer .... *iv*

Dedication .... *iv*

Preface .... *v*

Transportation Rules .... *vii*

Section I - The Essentials of Anatomy **11**

Section II - The Essentials of Sanitary Science **57**

Section III - The Essentials of Embalming **89**

Section IV - The Funeral Director **132**

Women as Embalmers 145

Dressing a Body 146

Dictionary of Anatomical Words and Phrases **148**

Disclaimer

Dedication

To the Funeral Directors and Embalmers of the United States and Canada who have so Generously Responded to My Feeble Efforts to Assist Them in Becoming More Competent in Their Profession, by the Purchase of My Former Works and by the Patronage They Have Given My School, I Dedicate This Little Volume.

Preface

In offering this little volume to the students of embalming and collateral sciences, I do so feeling that it will fill a want that has long been felt by the progressive embalmers of America. For several years past I have had frequent requests from students for a list of the questions most likely to be asked by the State Boards of Examiners, together with answers to the same. These requests became so frequent that I determined to write and publish a book containing all of the questions that could consistently be asked. To this end I have secured as many of the questions asked by examining boards as were obtainable — about six hundred — and to these have added many questions of my own, making in all about fourteen hundred, arranged them under appropriate headings, and answered them as briefly and concisely as possible.

Most of the questions I have printed exactly as asked by the examiners, but in a few of them, the meaning of which was very obscure, I have changed the wording slightly without changing the substance. Some of the questions having been asked several times with the phraseology slightly changed, have in substance been repeated. This has been done in order that the student may be well informed of the different manner of asking what is virtually the same question. The answers to the questions on anatomy have been given in the plainest and simplest language possible, and any anatomical terms used, the meaning of which might not be clear to the student, have been briefly and clearly defined in the dictionary contained in the work.

The answers to the questions on the care of special cases have been answered by the writer from a knowledge gained by personal experience in performing autopsies on bodies, dead of all kinds of diseases and causes, and by practical experience as an embalmer.

Most of the questions asked of the funeral director have been answered by myself from personal experience and observation, while some have been suggested by friends who are practical men of high standing in the profession. They will be found very valuable to the amateur funeral director and undertaker.

The questions on Sanitary Science, Disinfection and Disinfectants, have been arranged in order, and cover every question that can in fairness be asked by any examining board, and the answers have been so worded as

v

to convey to the student all the information necessary in the pursuit of that part of his calling relating to sanitation and disinfection, and to enable him to convince the board that he is possessed of a sufficient knowledge of sanitary science, so important a part of the education of the professional funeral director and embalmer.

Much more information can be gained by one day's study of this part of the work than can be obtained in a week by the perusal of the voluminous, complicated works called sanitary science, now on the market, some of which are clumsy copies wholly lacking in originality.

This work, together with "The Practical Embalmer," should do away with the necessity of taking a correspondence course of embalming, as there is no information that can possibly be obtained by such a course that is not much more briefly and plainly given in these books, and at less than one-fifth of the cost. Hoping that this, my third effort to benefit my brother embalmers, by placing before them my knowledge and experience in book form, may meet with their approval, I am,

Sincerely and fraternally yours,
A. JOHNSON DODGE.

Transportation Rules

Approved and Adopted by the American Association of General Baggage Agents, the Conference of State and Provincial Boards of Health, and the National Funeral Directors' Association

Rule 1. The transportation of bodies dead of small pox and bubonic plague, from one State, Territory, District or Province to another, is absolutely prohibited.

Rule 2. The transportation of bodies dead of Asiatic cholera, yellow fever, typhus fever, diphtheria (membraneous croup), scarlet fever (scarlatina, scarlet rash), erysipelas, glanders, anthrax or leprosy, shall not be accepted for transportation unless prepared for shipment by being thoroughly disinfected by (*a*) arterial and cavity injection with an approved disinfecting fluid; (*b*) disinfection and stopping of all orifices with absorbent cotton, and (*c*) washing the body with the disinfectant, all of which must be done by an embalmer holding a certificate as such, issued by the State or Provincial Board of Health, or other State or Provincial authority provided for by law.

After being disinfected as above, such bodies shall be enveloped in a layer of dry cotton not less than one inch thick, completely wrapped in a sheet securely fastened and encased in an air-tight zinc, copper or lead-lined coffin, or iron casket, all joints and seams hermetically seamed, and all enclosed in a strong, tight, wooden box, or the body being prepared for shipment by disinfecting and wrapping as above, may be placed in a strong coffin or casket, encased in an air-tight zinc, copper or tin-lined box, all joints and seams hermetically soldered.

For interstate transportation under this rule, Only embalmers holding a license issued or approved by the State or Provincial Boards of Health, or other State or Provincial authority provided by law, after examination, shall be recognized as competent to prepare such bodies for shipment.

Rule 3. The bodies of those dead of typhoid fever, puerperal fever, tuberculosis or measles, may be received for transportation when prepared for shipment by arterial and cavity injection with an approved disinfecting fluid, washing the exterior of the body with the same, and enveloping the entire body with a layer of cotton not less than one inch thick and all wrapped in a sheet securely fastened and encased in an air-tight metallic coffin or casket, or air-tight metal-lined box, provided that this shall apply only to bodies which can reach their destination within thirty hours from time of death. In all other cases, such bodies shall be prepared by a licensed embalmer holding a certificate as provided for in Rule 2, when air-tight sealing and bandaging with cotton may be dispensed with.

Rule 4. The bodies of those dead from any cause not stated in Rules 2 and 3 may be received for transportation when encased in a sound coffin or casket, and enclosed in a strong outside wooden box, provided they can reach their destination within thirty hours from time of death. If the body cannot reach its destination within thirty hours from the time of death, it must be prepared for shipment by arterial and cavity injection with an approved disinfecting fluid, washing the exterior of the body with the same and enveloping the entire body with a layer of dry cotton not less than one inch thick, and all wrapped in a sheet securely fastened and encased in an air-tight metallic coffin or casket or an airtight metal-lined box. But when the body has been prepared for shipment by being thoroughly disinfected by a licensed embalmer, as defined and directed in Rule 2, the air-tight sealing and bandaging with cotton may be dispensed with.

Rule 5. In the shipment of bodies dead from any disease named in Rule 2, such body must not be accompanied by persons or articles which have been exposed to the infection of the disease, unless certified by the health officer as having been properly disinfected.

Before selling ticket, agents should carefully examine the transit permit and note the name of the passenger in charge, and of any others proposing to accompany the body, and see that all necessary precautions have been taken to prevent the spread of the disease. The transit permit shall in such cases specifically state who is authorized by the health authorities to accompany the remains. In all cases where bodies are forwarded under Rule 2, notice must be sent by telegraph by the shipping embalmer to the health officer, or when there is no health officer, to other competent authority at destination, advising the date and train on which the body may be expected.

Rule 6. Every dead body must be accompanied by a person in charge, who must be provided with a passage ticket and also present a full first-class ticket marked "corpse" for the transportation of the body, and a transit permit showing physician's or coroner's certificate, name of deceased, date and hour of death, age, place of death, cause of death, and all other items of the standard certificate of death recommended by the American Public Health Association and adopted by the United States Census Bureau, as far as obtainable, including health officer's or registrar's permit for removal, whether a communicable or non-communicable disease, the point to which the body is to be shipped, and when death is caused by any of the diseases specified in Rule 2, the names of those authorized by the health authorities to accompany the body. Also the undertaker's certificate as to how the body has been prepared for shipment. The transit permit must be made in duplicate, and the signature of the physician or coroner, health officer and undertaker must be on both the original and duplicate copies. The undertaker's certificate and paster of the original shall be detached from the transit permit, and securely fastened on the end of the coffin box. All coffin boxes must be provided with at least four handles. The physician's certificate and transit permit shall be handed to the passenger in charge of the corpse. The whole duplicate copy shall be sent to the official in charge of the baggage department of the initial line, and by him to the secretary of the State or Provincial Board of Health of the State or Province from which said shipment is made.

Rule 7. When bodies are shipped by express a transit permit as described in Rule 6 must be made out in duplicate. The undertaker's certificate and paster of the original shall be detached from the transit permit and securely fastened on the coffin box. The physician's certificate and transit permit shall be attached to and accompany the express way bill covering the remains, and be delivered with the body at the point of destination to the person to whom it is consigned. The whole duplicate copy shall be sent by the forwarding express agent to the secretary of the State or Provincial Board of Health of the State or Province from which said shipment was made.

Rule 8. Every disinterred body, dead from any disease or cause, shall be treated as infectious or dangerous to the public health and shall not be accepted for transportation unless said removal has been approved by the State or Provincial health authorities having jurisdiction where such body is disinterred, and the consent of the health authorities of the locality to which the corpse is consigned has first been obtained; and all such disinterred remains, or the coffin or casket containing the same, must be wrapped in a woolen blanket thoroughly saturated with a 1-1000 solution of corrosive sublimate, and enclosed in a hermetically soldered zinc, tin, or copper-lined box. But bodies deposited in receiving vaults shall not be treated and considered the same as buried bodies when originally prepared by a licensed embalmer as defined in Rule 2, and as directed in Rule 2 or 3 (according to the nature of the disease causing death), provided shipment takes place within thirty days from time of death. The shipment of bodies prepared in the manner above directed by licensed embalmers from receiving vaults may be made within thirty days from the time of death without having to obtain permission from the health authorities of the locality to which the body is consigned. After thirty days the casket or coffin box containing said body must be enclosed in a hermetically soldered box.

Rule 9. All rules and parts of rules conflicting with these rules are hereby repealed.

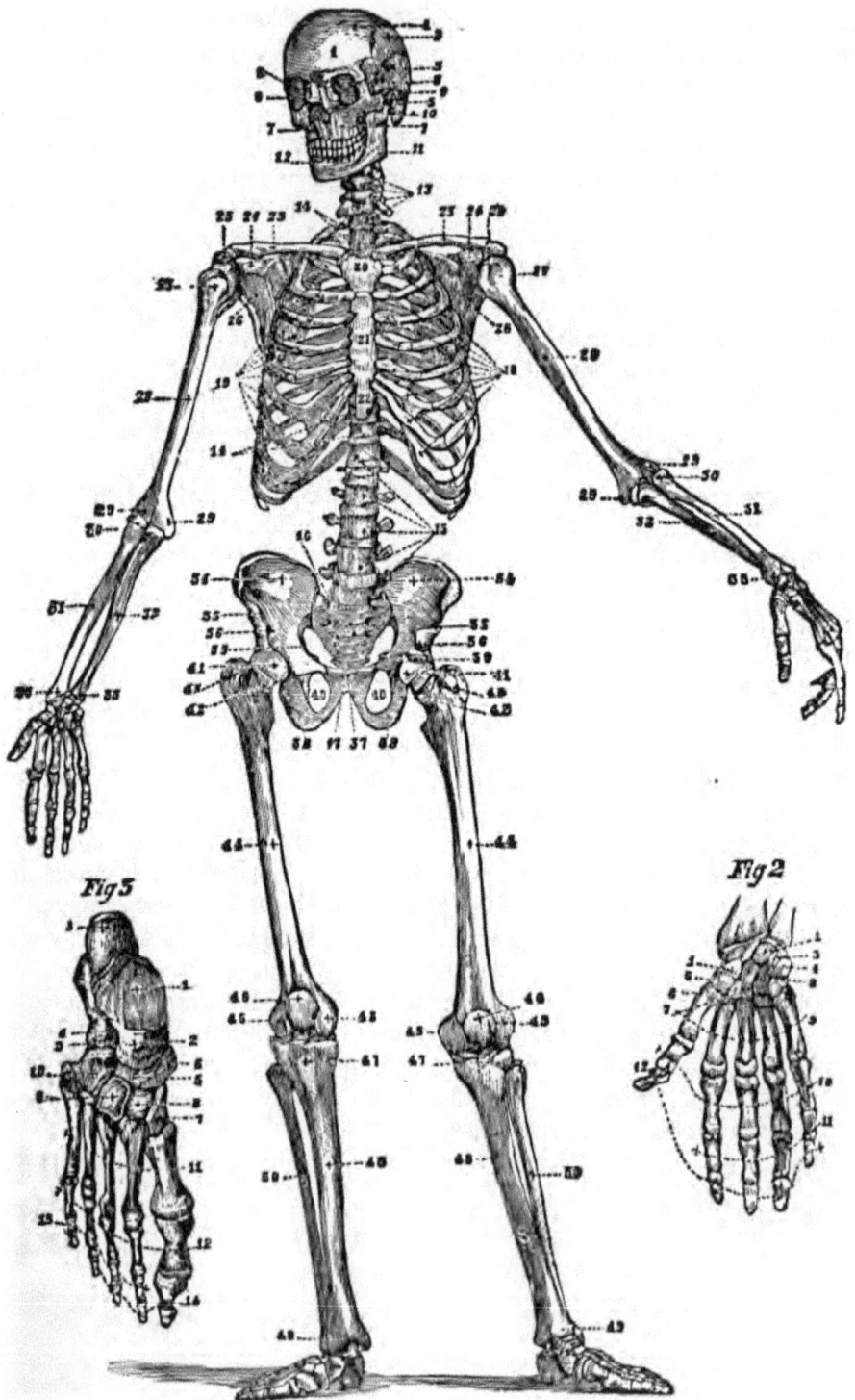

Section I - The Essentials of Anatomy

The Skeleton

Q. How many bones are there in the adult human body?

A. Excluding the bones of the ears, the teeth, the wormian and sesamoid bones, there are two hundred.

Q. How are bones classed?

A. They are classed as long, flat and irregular.

Q. Are bones vascular?

A. They are.

Q. What is meant by the word vascular?

A. Having vessels.

Q. What vessels are found in bones?

A. Arteries and veins, and some say lymphatics.

Q. How are the bones distributed?

A. Eight in the cranium, 14 in the face, 54 in the trunk, including the hyoid bone, 64 in the upper extremities and 60 in the lower extremities.

Q. Name the bones in the cranium.

A. One frontal, 2 parietal, 2 temporal, 1 occipital, 1 sphenoid and 1 ethmoid.

Q. Name the bones in the face.

A. Two malar, 2 nasal, 2 superior maxillary, 1 inferior maxillary, 2 palate, 2 lachrymal, 1 vomer and 2 turbinated.

Q. Name the bones of the trunk of the body above the pelvis.

A. The spinal column has 24 vertebrae, or joints (7 cervical in the neck, 12 dorsal in the back and 5 lumbar in the loins or lower portion of the back); the thorax has 14 true ribs in pairs, 6 false ribs in pairs, 4 floating ribs in pairs and 1 sternum.

The Human Skeleton

False Vertebrae

Bones of the Head, Trunk, Legs and Arms (Fig. 1.)

1. Frontal bone
2. Parietal bone.
3. Temporal bone.
4. Coronal suture.
5. Malar or cheek bone.
6. Nasal bones.
7. Superior maxillary, maxilla, or upper jawbone.
8. Orbits.
9. Side of occipital bone.
10. Condyloid process of mandible or lower jaw.
11. Angle of mandible.
12. Symphysis of mandible.
13. Four lower cervical vertebrae (7 In all)
14. Two upper and two lower dorsal vertebrae (12 in all).
15. Lumbar vertebrae (5 in number).
16. Sacrum. (false vertebrae)

17. Coccyx, the lower part hidden by the pubic bones. (false vertebrae)
18. Cartilages of ribs.
19. Ribs.
20. Manubrium of sternum or breast bone.
21. Mesosternum, or body of sternum.
22. Xiphisternum, metasternum, or ensiform process of sternum.
23. Clavicles, or collar bones.
24. Coracoid process of scapula (shoulder blade)
25. Acromion process of scapula.
26. Subscapular fossa, anterior surface.
27. Head of humerus or arm bone.
28. Body of humerus.
29. Condyles of humerus.
30. Head of radius or outer bone of forearm.
31. Body of radius.
32. Ulnar or inner bone of forearm.
33. Carpal ends of radius and ulna.
34. Internal iliac fossa.
35. Anterior superior process of ilium.
36. Anterior inferior process of ilium.
37. Pubic symphysis.
38. Tuberosity of ischium.
39. Brim of pelvis.
40. Obturator foramen.
41. Head of femur or thigh bone.
42. Neck of femur.
43. Great trochanter of femur.
44. Shaft of femur.
45. Condyles of femur.
46. Patella, or kneepan.
47. Head of tibia or thick bone on anterior and inner side of lee.
48. Shaft of tibia.
49. Lower extremity of tibia.
50. Fibula, or thin bone on external side of leg.

View of Palmar Surface of Right Hand and Wrist (Fig. 2.)

Bones of the carpus, or wrist: —
1. Scaphoid.
2. Semilunar.
3. Cuneiform.
4. Pisiform.
5. Trapezium.
6. Trapezoid.
7. Magnum.
8. Unciform.
9. Metacarpal bones of thumb and fingers.
10. First row of phalanges of thumb and fingers.
11. Second row or phalanges of fingers.
12. Third, or ungual, row of phalanges of fingers, and second, or ungual, phalanx of thumb.

Front View of Right Foot (Fig. 3.)

1, 3, 5, 7-10. Bones of the tarsus: —
1. Superior articulated surface of astragalus.
2. Anterior portion of astragalus.
3. Calcaneum, or heel bone.
4. Commencement of groove of interosseous ligament.
5. Scaphoid.
6. Tuberosity of scaphoid.
7. Internal cuneiform.
8. Middle cuneiform.
9. External cuneiform.
10. Cuboid.
11. Metatarsal bones.
12. First row of phalanges of toes.
13. Second row of phalanges of four outer toes.
14. Third, or ungual, row of phalanges of four outer toes and second, or ungual, phalanx of great toe.

Q. Name the bones in the pelvis.

A. The sacrum, coccyx and 2 ossa innominata.

Q. Name the bones of each upper extremity.

A. One scapula, 1 clavicle, 1 humerus, 1 radius, 1 ulna, 8 carpal, 5 metacarpal and 14 phalanges.

Q. Name the bones of each lower extremity.

A. One femur, i patella, i tibia, i 'fibula, 7 tarsal, 5 metatarsal and 14 phalanges.

Q. What is the function of the skeleton?

A. It is the framework on which the whole structure of the body is built.

Muscles, Fascia and Other Tissues

Q. What are muscles?

A. They are the organs of motion.

Q. Into how many classes are muscles divided?

A. Two; voluntary and involuntary.

Q. Which are the voluntary muscles?

A. Those under the control of the will.

Q. Which are involuntary muscles?

A. Those over which the will has no control.

Q. How do voluntary muscles move the bones?

A. By contraction. They are attached to the bones by white, shining bands, called tendons, and when the muscles contract the bone is lifted or moved as directed by the will.

Q. Describe the voluntary muscles.

A. They are composed of long, soft, fleshy fibres, lying parallel one with the other and bound together with a thin cellular membrane into little bundles, and these into larger bundles, until the whole muscle is formed.

Q. What is the appearance of the voluntary muscles?

A. They are of the reddish color characteristic of the flesh; they are the lean flesh of the body.

Q. Of what interest are the muscles to the embalmer?

A. They serve as guides in locating the vessels used in embalming the body and in drawing the blood. They also constitute the greater portion of the body which we are called upon to preserve and disinfect.

Q. Name a few of the involuntary muscles.

A. The heart and the walls of the arteries, the stomach and the walls of the intestines.

Q. What is the fascia?

A. A dense, fibrous membrane, serving as a wrap or bandage, hence the name.

Q. How is the fascia classed?

A. As superficial and deep.

Q. What is the function of the superficial fascia, and where is it located?

A. Its function is to protect the superficial veins and nerves which lie between its folds. It is located just beneath the skin and extends over almost the whole surface of the body.

Q. What is the function of the deep fascia?

A. To wrap up and bind down. It wraps up the arteries, veins and nerves, and binds down the muscles.

Q.. What is the meaning of the word tissue?

A. Most of the substance of the body is called tissue, particularly the flesh.

Q. Name some of the tissues.

A. Muscular, fibrous, areolar and connective tissue.

Q. What is meant by areolar tissue?

A. Fatty tissue found between the skin and the muscles, connective cellular tissue.

Q. What is meant by muscular tissue?

A. That substance of which the muscles are composed, the largest portion being what is known as lean flesh.

Q. How many muscles in the human body?

A. About 500.

Q. Is the study of the muscles a necessary part of the education of the embalmer?

A. It is not; a superficial knowledge, particularly of those muscles which serve as guides to the arteries is all that is necessary.

Q. What is the subcutaneous tissue?

A. Subcutaneous cellular tissue lies beneath the skin. It is continuous over most of the body.

Q. la this tissue liable to cause trouble to the embalmer?

A. Yes; it sometimes decomposes rapidly, causing what is known as tissue gas and slipping of the epidermis.

Q. What is the skin?

A. It is an elastic membrane, acting as a protection or covering for the deeper tissues of the body. It consists of two layers, the derma or cutis vera (true skin), and the epidermis or outer skin, also called the scarf skin or cuticle.

Q. Describe the epidermis.

A. It is a non-vascular, shell-like substance, designed to protect the blood vessels and nerves of the true skin. It is thickest on the exposed parts of the body and more soft and thin on the less exposed parts.

Q. Are the nails and the hair formed from the true or scarf skin?

A. They are an outgrowth of the cuticle.

The Cavities of the Body

Q. How many cavities in the trunk of the body?

A. Two; the thoracic and abdominal.

Q. What other cavities are there in the body?

A. The cavity of the cranium or cerebro-spinal cavity, the cavity of the pelvis, and the serous or minor cavities in the thorax, called the right and left pleural and the mediastinal cavities.

Q. What forms the cavity of the cranium?

A. The bones of the skull.

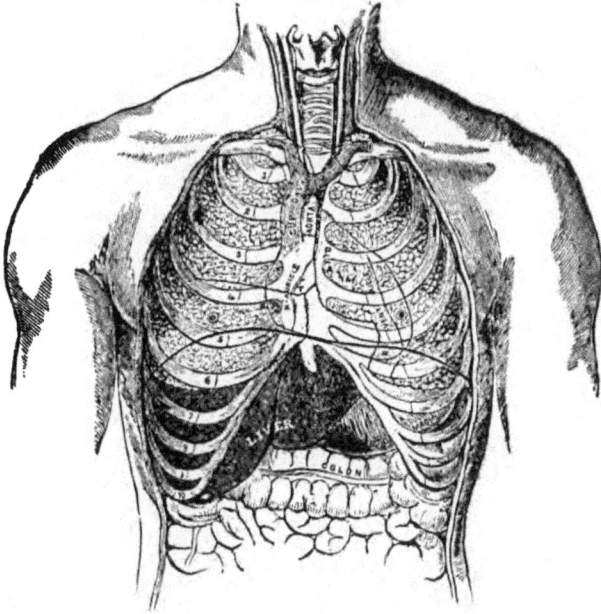

Front View of Thorax, Showing Viscera

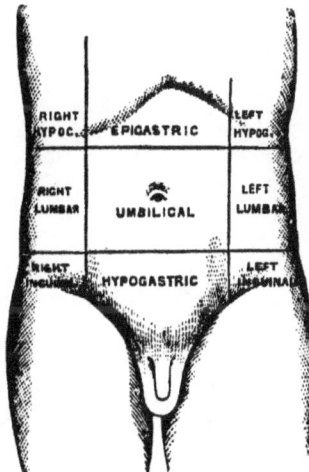

Divisions of the Abdominal Cavity

Q. Describe the thorax.

A. It is a bony, cartilaginous cage, formed behind by the dorsal portion of the spinal column and the commencing ribs, laterally by the ribs, in front by

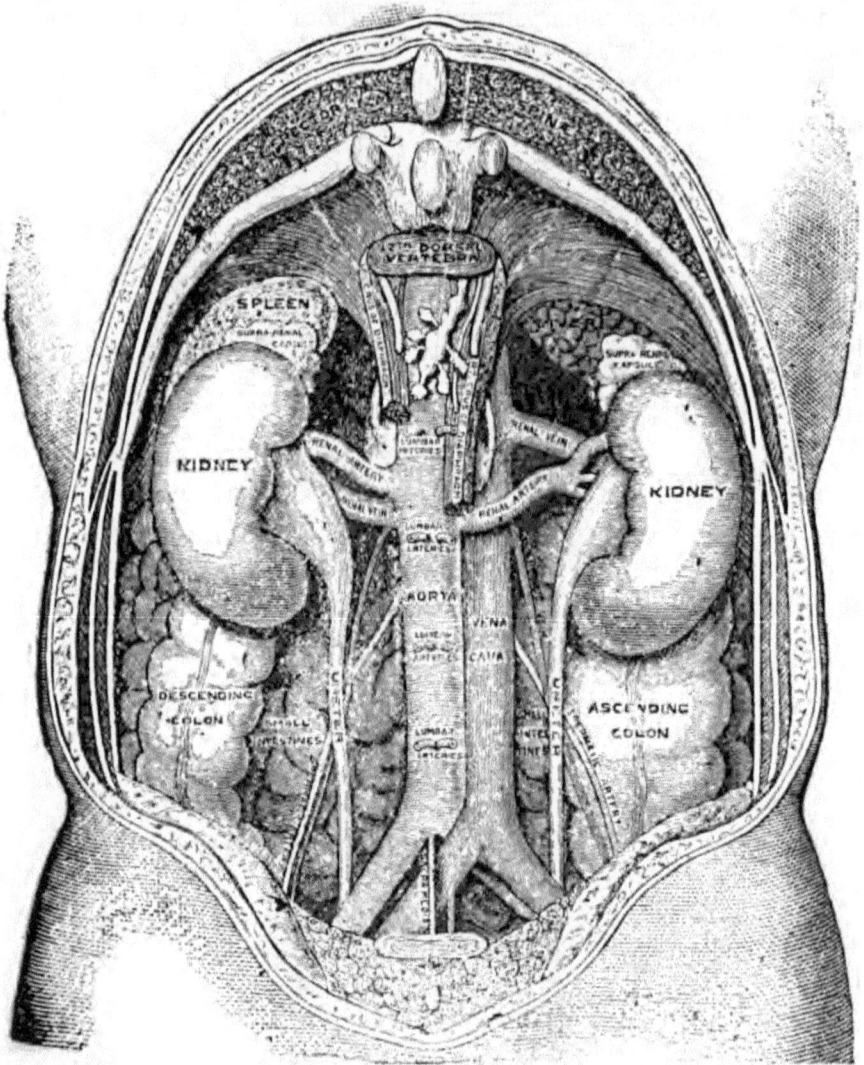

Back View of Abdomen. Showing Viscera and Large Vessels

the sternum or breast bone and the costal cartilage, above by the neck and below by the diaphragm. It is conical in shape, being wider below than above, and wider from side to side than from front to back. It is divided by a membrane, called the pleura, into three minor cavities, the right and left pleural, and the mediastinum.

Q. Describe the abdominal cavity.

A. It is the largest cavity in the body, is oval in shape, bounded below by the brim of the pelvis and above by the diaphragm, on the sides and in the front by the lower ribs and the abdominal muscles, and behind by the spinal column and the muscles of the back.

Q. Into what regions is the abdominal cavity divided?

A. It is divided into nine regions by four imaginary lines, two horizontal ones, one between the cartilages of the ninth ribs and another between the crests of the ileum, and two vertical ones, extending from the points of the cartilage of the eighth ribs to the centre of Poupart's ligaments. These regions are called right hypochondriac, right lumbar, right inguinal, epigastric, umbilical, hypogastric, left hypochondriac, left lumbar, left inguinal.

Q. Describe the peritoneum.

A. The peritoneum is a serous membrane, which covers the bowels and wholly or partially invests all of the viscera contained in the abdominal cavity. This membrane is very complicated and hard to understand in all its different aspects. It is a closed sac, one fold of which, called the parietal invests the posterior walls of the abdomen, and the other, called the visceral, most of the viscera.

Q. Describe the pelvic cavity.

A. It is formed by the union of the pelvic bones with the abdominal muscles. On account of its resemblance to a dish it is often called the pelvic basin.

Q. Describe the pleural cavities.

A. They are formed by a double-fold membrane, called the pleura, one of which, called the parietal, lines the posterior walls of the thorax; and the other, known as the visceral fold, invests the lungs. The interspaces between the two folds of this membrane are called the pleural cavities.

Q. Are the pleural cavities separate or connected?

A. There is no open connection between the right and left pleural cavities.

Q. What is the mediastinum?

A. The space in the middle of the chest, between the pleurae.

Q. What is the cavity of the pericardium?

A. The interior of the membranous sac enclosing the heart.

Q. What is meant by the peritoneal cavity?

A. As already stated, the peritoneum is a membrane forming a closed sac, one fold lining the posterior walls of the abdomen, the other fold investing the viscera; the interspace between the folds is often called the peritoneal cavity. There is, however, little or no difference between the peritoneal and abdominal cavities.

Q. Name the principal viscera in the thoracic cavity.

A. The heart and lungs.

Q. Name the principal viscera in the cavity of the abdomen.

A. The liver, stomach, spleen, pancreas, gall bladder, large and small intestines and the kidneys.

Q. Name the viscera in the cavity of the pelvis.

A. The bladder and rectum in the male. The bladder, womb and rectum in the female.

Visceral Anatomy

Q. What is visceral anatomy?
A. The science of the structure of the viscera, or organs located in the serous cavities.
Q. Name six visceral organs.
A. Brain, heart, liver, spleen, stomach and pancreas.
Q. What is the diaphragm and where is it located?
A. It is a muscular membrane situated between the thoracic and abdominal cavities, forming a roof for the last named cavity and a floor for the lungs.
Q. What organs are in contact with the diaphragm?
A. The heart, lungs, liver, stomach and spleen.
Q. How many openings in the diaphragm? Name them.
A. Three. The oesophageal and the aortic openings, and an opening for the inferior vena cava; the thoracic duct also passes through the diaphragm.
Q. What are the organic viscera of the human body?
A. All organs contained in the serous cavities of the body, including the suprarenal capsules and the absorbent glands.
Q. Name the organic tissues of the cranial, thoracic and abdominal cavities.
A. The cranial cavity, the brain and its membrane; the thoracic cavity, the heart and lungs, part of the trachea, the bronchi, part of the oesophagus, the superior vena cava and part of the inferior; the abdominal cavity, the liver, stomach, spleen, pancreas, gall bladder, large and small intestines, the kidneys and the suprarenal capsules. Some authorities would include the urinary bladder and the uterus in females, but this is properly pelvic viscera.

The Brain

Q. Describe the brain.
A. The brain is the organ of intelligence, situated in the cavity of the cranium. It is a soft, pulpy mass of a whitish color inside, and a greyish color on the outside. It has three membranes; the outer, which is called the dura mater, lining the skull and investing the brain. This membrane also acts as a partition wall, dividing the brain into sections, the principal of which are the right and the left hemispheres. The inner membrane is called the pia mater. It is soft, delicate and very vascular. Between these two membranes is spread a third, which is extremely delicate, resembling a cobweb. The brain is divided into four parts; the cerebrum or large brain, the cerebellum or small brain, the medulla oblongata and pons varolii. The average weight of the brain in the male is from forty-eight to fifty-two ounces. It is about five ounces lighter in the female.

The Lungs

Q. Describe the lungs.

A. The lungs are the organs of respiration and also the organs in which the blood is purified. They are situated one on either side in the thoracic cavity. The apex of each lung is behind and a little above the collar bone. The base of the lungs rest on the convex surface of the diaphragm. The right lung has three lobes and the left but two, and the right is much wider and stronger than the other, nature having made this provision in order to accommodate the heart, which inclines to the left. The tissue of which the lungs are composed is light, spongy and elastic, having a multitude of air cells into which open the bronchial tubes. Each lung is invested by a delicate serous membrane called the pleura. The weight of the lungs in the male adult is about forty-four ounces. In the female they are several ounces lighter.

Q. Name the blood vessels of the lungs.

A. The pulmonary arteries and pulmonary veins, the bronchial arteries and the bronchial veins.

Q. What is the vital capacity of the lungs?

A. They may contain about two hundred and twelve to two hundred and thirty cubic inches of air at a forced inspiration.

Q. How much air is taken into the lungs at each respiration?

A. About twenty cubic inches, or one-third of a pint.

Q. How much air passes and repasses through the average lungs in twenty-four hours?

A. About three hundred and fifty cubic feet.

Q. How many air cells do the lungs contain?

A. Authorities differ, giving the number as from three to eight millions.

Q. How are air cells formed?

A. By a membranous partition, called a septa.

Q. What is the size of the air cells of the lungs?

A. From one two-hundredths to one-seventieth of an inch in diameter.

Q. What structure surrounds each lung and lines the posterior walls of the thorax to form a cavity?

A. A membraneous sac called the pleura.

The Trachea

Q. Describe the trachea.

A. The trachea or wind-pipe, is formed of cartilaginous rings and .an elastic membrane. The rings are intended to keep the tubes constantly open for the passage of air; they do not form a circle, however, as that part of the trachea resting on the oesophagus is composed almost wholly of the membrane which also binds the rings together and completes the sides of the tube. The trachea is about four and one-half inches long, descending from the larynx (the organ of voice) to its bifurcation into the right and left bronchus, which enter the lungs where they divide and subdivide into the bronchial tubes. The trachea and its divisions and subdivisions are kept constantly moist by a mucus secreted by the glands which are found all along the membrane lining the tube.

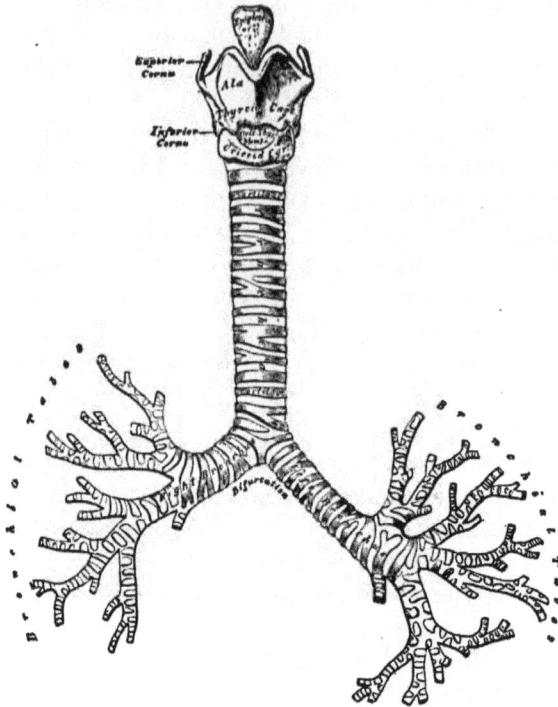

The Trachea and Bronchi

The Heart

Q. Describe the heart, giving size, shape, weight, location, chambers, valves and movements.

A. The heart is a hollow muscular organ, in shape an inverted cone. It is situated in the mediastinal space, between the right and left lungs. Its base is nearly on a line with the lower border of the third costal cartilage. Its apex is about two and one-half inches to the left of the sterum, between the fifth and sixth ribs. The two sides, the right being the venous and the left the arterial side of the heart, are divided by a muscular wall called a septum. The heart is further divided into chambers or cavities called auricles and ventricles. This again is accomplished by a lighter wall also called a septum. The valves which guard the entrance from the right auricle to the right ventricle are called the tricuspid valves. Those which guard the entrance from the left auricle to the left ventricle are called the bicuspid or mitral valves. The valves located at the entrance to the pulmonary artery are called semilunar pulmonary valves, those at the entrance to the great aorta, semilunar aortic valves.

The heart is five inches long, three and one-half inches wide, two and one-half inches thick, and weighs from nine and one-half to twelve ounces. The normal movement of the heart is seventy-two pulsations per minute.

Q. Why are the semilunar valves so called?

A. Because they are in the shape of a half moon (semi-one-half; lunar, the moon).

Q. Why are the tricuspid valves so called?

A. Because they have three points or cusps.

Q. Why are the mitral valves so called?

A. Because they are shaped like a mitre.

Q. Name the blood vessels of the heart.

A. The coronary arteries and the cardiac veins.

Q. How is the right auricle of the heart connected with the right ventricle?

A. By the auriculo-ventricular orifice, which is guarded by the tricuspid valve.

Q. What structure or tissue surrounds the heart and forms a cavity?

A. The pericardium.

Q. What is the function of the heart?

A. It performs the function of a force pump, to force the blood through the circulatory vessels.

Q. Has the heart more than one function?

A. In a certain sense it has. The right side receives the venous blood from the veins and forces it to the lungs for purification. The left side receives the pure blood from the pulmonary veins and forces it into the arteries which convey it to the tissues for nourishment. However, if asked what is the function of 'the heart, the answer should be to force the blood through the circulatory system.

Q. What is the position of the heart relative to the lungs?

A. It lies between the lungs, the base being in the centre, the apex inclining to the left and in contact with the left lung.

The Liver

Q. Describe the liver, giving location, size, weight and function.

A. The liver is the largest gland in the body. It is situated on the right side of the body just below the diaphragm, its left lobe overlapping the stomach. It is from ten to twelve inches in length, from six to seven inches wide and about three inches thick. Its weight is about four and one-half pounds. Its principal function is the secretion of bile.

Q. How many lobes has the liver? Name them.

A. Five; the right and left, and three minor lobes known as the lobulus quadratus, caudatus and lobulus spigelii.

Q. How many fissures has the liver?

A. Five; they separate the lobes.

Q. Name the vessels of the liver.

A. Portal vein, hepatic arteries, hepatic veins, hepatic ducts and lymphatics.

Q. To what extent has the liver been known to enlarge?

A. To the weight of twenty pounds or more.

Q. Is this enlargement of any interest to the embalmer?

A. It is, as an enlarged liver needs special treatment.

The Spleen

Q. Describe the spleen.

A. It is a small glandular organ situated on the left side of the body, below the stomach and above the left kidney. It is composed of soft, brittle tissue and is very vascular. It varies in size in different individuals, being generally about four inches in length by three in width.

Q. Name the blood vessels of the spleen.

A. The splenic artery and the splenic vein.

Q. What is the weight of the spleen? Give its function.

A. Its weight is from five to eight ounces. The function of the spleen is not yet positively known.

Q. Is the spleen liable to enlargement, and if so, to what extent?

A. It has been known to reach the weight of twenty pounds.

Q. Is this of interest to embalmers?

A. Yes, as in this condition the spleen cannot be preserved by arterial embalming and other methods must be resorted to.

The Kidneys

Q. Describe the kidneys, giving location, size, weight and function.

A. The kidneys are two in number, situated one on either side of the spinal column, in the right and left lumbar regions. They are tubular glands, four inches long, two wide and one thick. Their weight is from four and one-half to six ounces each. Their function is to secrete urine.

Q. Name the vessels that convey blood to and from the kidneys.

A. The renal arteries and veins.

Q. How is the urine conveyed to the bladder?

A. Through convoluted tubes, called ureters.

The Alimentary Canal

Q. What is the alimentary canal?

A. The food passage from mouth to anus.

Q. Name its different parts or divisions.

A. The principal divisions are the mouth, pharynx or throat, oesophagus or gullet, stomach and small and large intestines.

Q. Name the minor divisions of the intestines.

A. The small intestine is divided into three portions; doudenum, jejunum and ileum. The large intestine has six divisions; caecum, ascending, transverse and descending colon, sigmoid flexure and rectum.

Q. How long is the alimentary canal?

A. About twenty-eight feet.

Q. How long is the intestinal canal?

A. About twenty-five feet.

Q. Describe the pharynx.

A. It is a conical, muscular sac, about four and one-half inches long and wider above than below, its narrowest part being at its termination in the oesophagus. It has three coats, fibrous, muscular and mucous, and seven openings, two posterior nares (nostrils), two Eustachian tubes, the mouth, larynx and oesophagus.

Q. Describe the oesophagus.

A. It is a muscular tube nine inches in length, and having three coats. It connects the pharynx with the stomach. Its function is to convey food to the stomach.

Q. Name and describe the coats of the oesophagus.

A. The inner, mucous, a thin membrane; the middle, cellular, composed of cellular tissue, and the outer, muscular, made up of fibrous muscular tissue.

Q. Describe the stomach, giving location, capacity, size, weight and function.

A. The stomach is the principal organ of digestion, and the most distended part of the alimentary canal. It is located in the upper portion of the abdominal cavity in what is known as the epigastric regions, but extends almost entirely across the body, and is in close contact with the diaphragm. It is from ten to twelve inches in length, and from four to six inches in diameter when moderately distended, but varies in size more than any other organ of the body, its capacity being from one to three quarts. Its weight when empty is said to be from five to eight ounces.

Q. Which is the larger end of the stomach?

A. That on the left side, called the cardiac or splenic end.

Q. Which is the smaller end?

A. That on the right side, called the pyloric end.

Q. Are there any valves connected with the stomach?

A. Yes, one, the pyloric valve. It is situated in the pylorus at its entrance to the duodenum.

Q. How many coats has the stomach?

A. Three; the inner, mucous; the middle, muscular; and the outer, peritoneal or serous.

Q. How many openings has the stomach?

A. Two; the oesophageal, opening in, and the pyloric, opening out.

Q. What is the next link in the alimentary canal?

A. The duodenum.

Q. How long is it?
A. Twelve inches long.
Q. How long is the jejunum?
A. About seven feet long.
Q. How long is the ileum?
A. About twelve feet.
Q. Into what does the ileum open?
A. Into the caecum.
Q. Are there any valves connected with this opening?
A. Yes, the ileo-caecal valve.
Q. Where is the vermiform appendix?
A. Attached to the caecum.
Q. How many coats have the intestines?
A. Four; serous, muscular, cellular and mucous.
Q. How long is the small intestine?
A. About twenty feet.
Q. How long is the large intestine?
A. About five feet.
Q. Name the blood vessels of the intestines. **A.** The superior and inferior mesenteric arteries, and the mesenteric veins.

The Pancreas

Q. Describe the pancreas.
A. It is a gland about seven or eight inches long and two wide. It is situated behind the stomach, extending from the pylorus to the spleen. The wider or pyloric end is called the head of the pancreas, while that part near the spleen is more narrow and is called the tail. Its function is to secrete pancreatic juice.

The Gall Bladder

Q. Describe the gall bladder.
A. It is a small, pear-shaped sac attached to the right lobe of the liver. It serves as a reservoir for the bile, its capacity being about one and one-half ounces.

The Pelvic Viscera

Q. Give a brief description of the womb.
A. It is a small muscular organ, located in the pelvic cavity, between the bladder and the rectum. In its virgin state it is very small, being only about three inches in length, two in breadth and one in thickness, and weighing about two and one-half ounces. It is the organ of child bearing, and in pregnancy will distend until its upper portions may be found in the epigastric region.
Q. By what other name is the womb known?

A. It is often called the uterus.

Q. Describe the urinary bladder.

A. It is a small sac or bag, located in the pelvis, just behind the pubes or pubic bone.

Q. What is its function?

A. It is a reservoir for the urine, and in its normal state holds about one pint. On account of stoppage of the water, it has been known to distend until it held twelve pints.

THE VASCULAR SYSTEM

Q. Of what does the vascular system consist?

A. The vascular system includes the heart, arteries, capillaries, veins and lympathics.

Q. What is the difference between the circulatory and vascular systems?

A. The circulatory system is the blood-vascular system, and does not include the lymphatics; the vascular system is more comprehensive; it includes both the circulatory system and the lymphatic, or water-vascular system.

Q. What is the function of the heart?

A. To force the blood through the circulatory system by the contraction of its muscular walls.

Q. What is the difference between the contraction of the auricles and that of the ventricles of the heart?

A. The contraction of the ventricles takes place simultaneously from all sides, so that the pressure within is equal in every direction. The auricles contract peristaltically from the opening of the supplying vessels toward the orifice leading to the ventricles.

Q. Which have the thicker walls, the ventricles or the auricles?

A. The ventricles, owing to the greater force they are required to exert.

Q. What is the function of the right auricle?

A. To force the blood through the tricuspid valves into the right ventricle.

Q. What is the function of the left auricle of the heart?

A. To force the blood through the bicuspid or mitral valves into the left ventricle.

Q. What is the function of the right ventricle of the heart?

A. To force the blood through the semilunar pulmonary valves into the pulmonary arteries and along those vessels to the lungs.

Q. What is the function of the left ventricle of the heart?

A. To force the blood through the semilunar aortic valves into the great aorta, and through its branches and subbranches, assisted by the contraction of the arterial walls, to the capillaries.

Q. Has the right side of the heart any suction power enabling it to aid in the return of the blood through the veins?

A. No; it was formerly supposed to have, but modern research has disproved that theory.

Q. What is the function of the valves of the heart?

A. To prevent the regurgitation of the blood from the ventricles to the auricles or from the arteries back into the ventricles.

The Arteries

Q. What are arteries?

A. Tubular vessels, whose function is the conveyance of blood from both ventricles of the heart to all parts of the body or to the capillaries.

Q. How many kinds of arteries are there in the body?

A. Two, systemic and pulmonary.

Q. Of what do the systemic arteries consist?

A. The aorta, the great trunk artery of the body, and all of its branches and sub-branches.

Q. What are the pulmonary arteries?

A. Vessels which originating in the right ventricle of the heart, extend upwards about two and one-half inches and divide into the right and left pulmonary arteries, which convey venous blood to the lungs for purification.

Q. Where do arteries originate?

A. At the ventricles of the heart.

Q. Where do they terminate?

A. They terminate in the capillaries.

Q. Where does the great aorta originate?

A. In the left ventricle of the heart.

Q. How is the aorta divided?

A. It is divided into the arch, the thoracic and the abdominal aorta.

Q. What is the thoracic aorta?

A. All that portion of the vessel below the third dorsal vetebra and above the diaphragm.

Q. What is the abdominal aorta?

A. All that portion below the diaphragm and above the fourth lumba vertebra.

Q. How many coats have arteries? Describe them.

A. Three, an internal or serous coat, a middle coat composed of muscular and elastic tissue, and an external coat composed of fibrous connective tissue. The last named is the only coat containing blood vessels.

Q. How many branches arise from the arch of the aorta?

A. Five; the innominate, left common carotid, left subclavian, and two coronary.

Q. Name the principal branches of the thoracic aorta.

A. The intercostal, bronchial, oesophageal, and posterior mediastinal.

Q. Give the principal branches of the abdominal aorta.

A. The coeliac axis, the superior and inferior mesenteric, phrenic, renal, supra-renal, spermatic and lumbar arteries.

Q. At what point does the abdominal aorta terminate?

A. Opposite the fourth lumbar vertebra.

Q. Into what does it divide?

A. Into the right and left common iliac arteries.

Q. Describe the innominate artery.

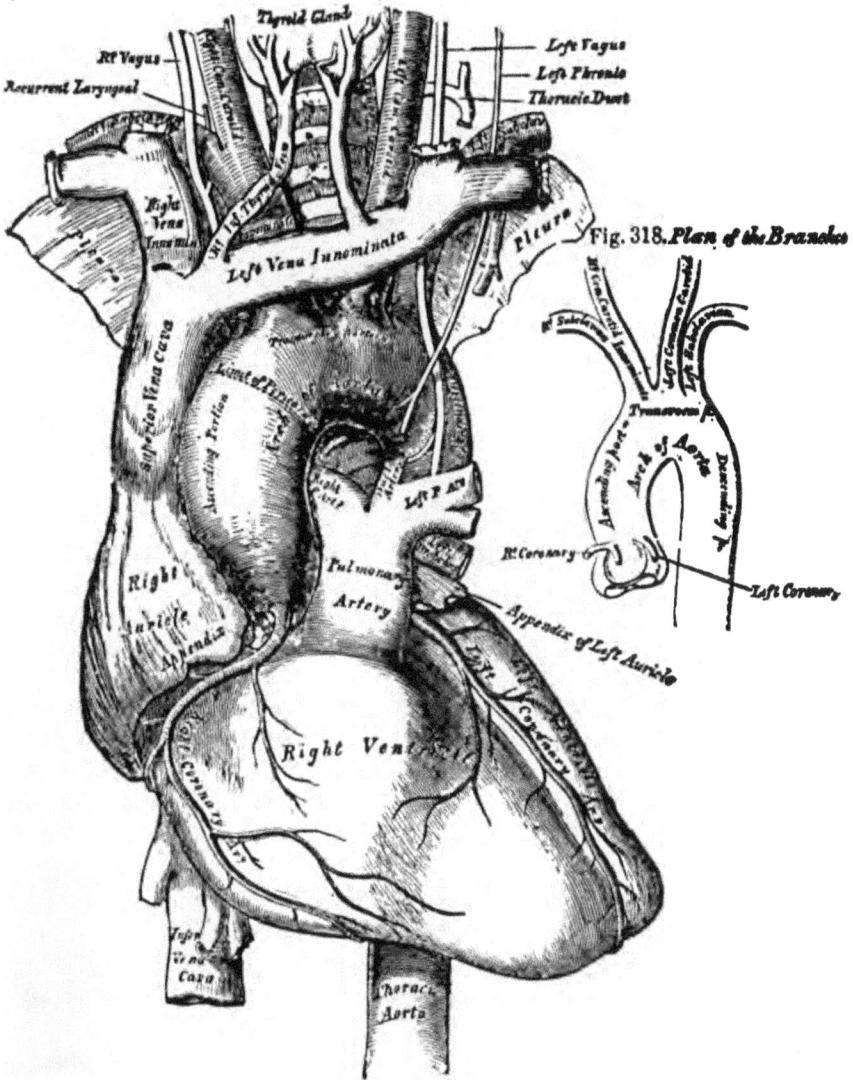

Fig. 318. *Plan of the Branches*

The Arch of the Aorta and Its Branches

A. The innominate artery rises from the right side of the arch of aorta and extends upward from one and one-half to two inches to the junction of the sternum and clavicle, where it divides into the right common carotid and right subclavian arteries.

Q. Describe the right common carotid artery.

A. The right common carotid artery ascends obliquely between the trachea and sterno mastoid muscle until directly opposite the Adam's apple, where it divides into the external and internal carotid arteries.

Q. Describe the left common carotid artery.

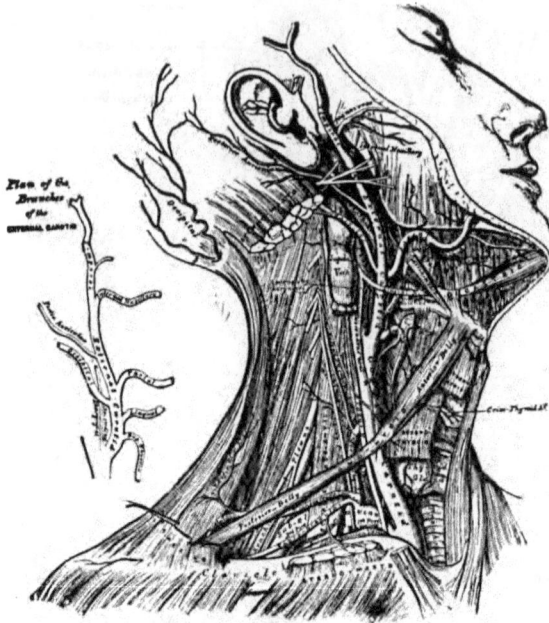

Right Side of Neck and Face, showing the Arteries of the Neck

A. The left common carotid artery differs from the right only in its origin, which is at the anterior middle of the arch of the aorta instead of from the innominate artery (there being no innominate artery on the left side of the arch). The common carotid arteries usually have no branches, but they occasionally give origin to the vertebral, and sometimes to the superior and inferior thyroid.

Q. Describe the external and internal carotid arteries.

A. The external and internal carotid arteries, the divisions of the common carotids, have eight branches each, some of which it is well for the embalmer to be acquainted with, as they convey the fluid to very important parts of the body. The branches of the external carotid arteries are the superior thyroid, lingual, facial, internal maxillary, temporal, occipital, posterior auricular and ascending pharyngeal. The first important branch of the external carotid artery is the facial, often very appropriately called the tortuous facial artery. It arises just below the lower jaw, extends upward and passes over the cheek to the angle of the mouth, giving off branches in its passage. It is very tortuous and in many places very superficial. When the body is being injected rapidly, this artery and its branches may be seen to enlarge to a considerable extent.

The internal carotid artery, like the external, commences at the division of the common carotid, and running perpendicularly upward passes through the carotid canal and enters the skull. Still passing upward it enters the cavernous sinus, pierces the dura mater and divides into its terminal branches. This vessel supplies the anterior portion of the brain, the eye and its appendages. It is remarkable for its many curvatures, which are probably intended to lessen the rapidity of the current of blood in its passage to the brain. The internal carotid artery, like the external, has eight branches, four of which supply the brain, the balance supplying the petrous and cavernous portions of the head.

Q. Describe the circle of Willis.

A. The branches of the internal carotid and the vertebral arteries anastomose at the base of the brain in such a manner as to form a sort of circle, called the circle of Willis. It is formed in front by the anterior cerebral and the anterior communicating arteries, on each side by the trunk of the internal carotid and the posterior communicating, behind by the posterior cerebral and the point of the basilar. By this anastomosis, the circulation of the brain is equalized. It has long been taught that it is by piercing this circle that an arterial circulation is obtained by the so-called needle process of embalming. The fallacy of this teaching will be shown later on.

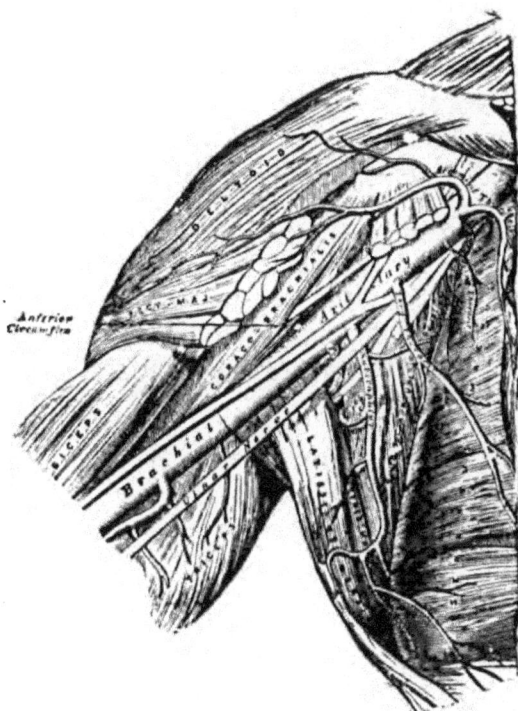

The Axillary and Brachial Arteries

Q. Describe the subclavian arteries.

A. The right subclavian artery arises from the innominate artery, at its bifurcation at the junction of the sternum and collar bone. The left subclavian arises from the highest part of the arch of the aorta. On the right side this artery ascends obliquely outward from its origin. On the left it ascends vertically to the same point. They then pass outward, across the roots of the neck, under the clavicle or collar bone to the lower border of the first rib, where they enter the axillary space and become the axillary arteries.

The branches of the subclavian artery are four in number, the vertebral being its largest branch, and the only one in which the embalmer need be particularly interested. This branch enters the interior of the skull, through the foramen magnum, at the back of the head, and forms a part of the circle of Willis by anastomosing with the internal carotid artery.

Q. Describe the axillary artery.

A. The axillary artery is a continuation of the subclavian; commences at the termination of the latter vessel and extends outward towards the arm for about two inches, where it becomes the brachial artery. The branches of the axillary artery are seven in number, none of which are of any particular interest to the embalmer.

Q. Describe the brachial artery.

A. The brachial artery is a continuation of the axillary; it commences at the termination of that vessel and extends along the base of the biceps muscle to a point half an inch below the bend of the elbow, where it terminates by dividing into the radial and ulnar arteries. This vessel is accompanied by its venae coraites and the median nerve, all of which are enclosed in a sheath. The branches of this artery are the superior profunda, nutrient, inferior profunda, anastomotica magna and the muscular branches.

Q. Describe the radial artery.

A. The radial artery, the smaller of the two divisions of the brachial, commences at the bifurcation of that vessel, about one-half inch below the bend of the elbow, and extends on the radial or thumb side of the forearm between the two muscles to the wrist, where in life the pulse is usually felt. The radial artery is superficial in almost its entire extent, but more particularly in the lower third of its course. This vessel has no veins except venae comites, which are very

Superficial Anatomy of the Radial Artery. Showing the Muscular Guides

small, and give the embalmer no trouble. The radial artery has twelve branches, none of which are of any importance to embalmers.

Q. Describe the ulnar artery.

A. The ulnar artery, the other division of the brachial, is the larger of the two, but, as it is much more deeply seated and harder to secure, it is seldom used by embalmers. It can, however, be used to advantage if raised in the lower part of the wrist. This artery commences at the bifurcation of the brachial and passes along the inner side of the forearm obliquely inward to the commencement of its lower half. It then runs along its ulnar border to the wrist on the little finger side of the arm. It can be found between the tendons of the muscles, just external to the flexor carpi ulnaris muscle.

Q. Describe the palmar arch.

A. The superficial palmar arch is that part of the ulnar artery lying in the palm of the hand, and anastomosing with branches from the radial. It gives off four branches, the digital, to the sides of the fingers, except the inside of the index finger, which is supplied by another branch. The deep palmar arch is formed by the palmar portion of the radial artery anastomosing with the deep or communicating branch of the ulnar. It gives off six branches, none of which are of any importance to the embalmer.

Q. Describe the coronary arteries.

A. The coronary arteries are two in number, the right and the left. They arise from the aorta, behind the semilunar valves, and wind through the ventricular grooves of the heart, the left artery in front, to supply the tissues of that organ.

Q. Describe the bronchial arteries.

A. The bronchial arteries supply the lungs with pure blood. These arteries vary in number and origin. Those from the right side arise from the intercostal artery, or from a common stock with the left bronchial from the front of the aorta. These are the nutrient vessels of the lungs and are the first arteries to carry the fluid to those organs when the body is being injected.

Q. Describe the oesophageal arteries.

A. The oesophageal arteries are the nutrient vessels of the oesophagus. They are four or five in number, and arise from the front of the tho-

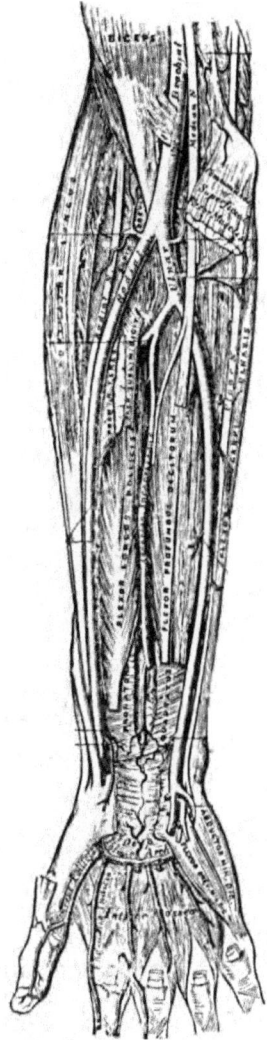

Deep Anatomy, Showing the Radial and Ulnar Arteries, and the Median Nerve

racic aorta, pass obliquely downward to the oesophagus, anastomosing and forming a chain along that tube.

Q. Describe the intercostal arteries.

A. The intercostal arteries arise from the back part of the aorta. They are usually ten in number on each side, and are distributed to the intercostal muscles.

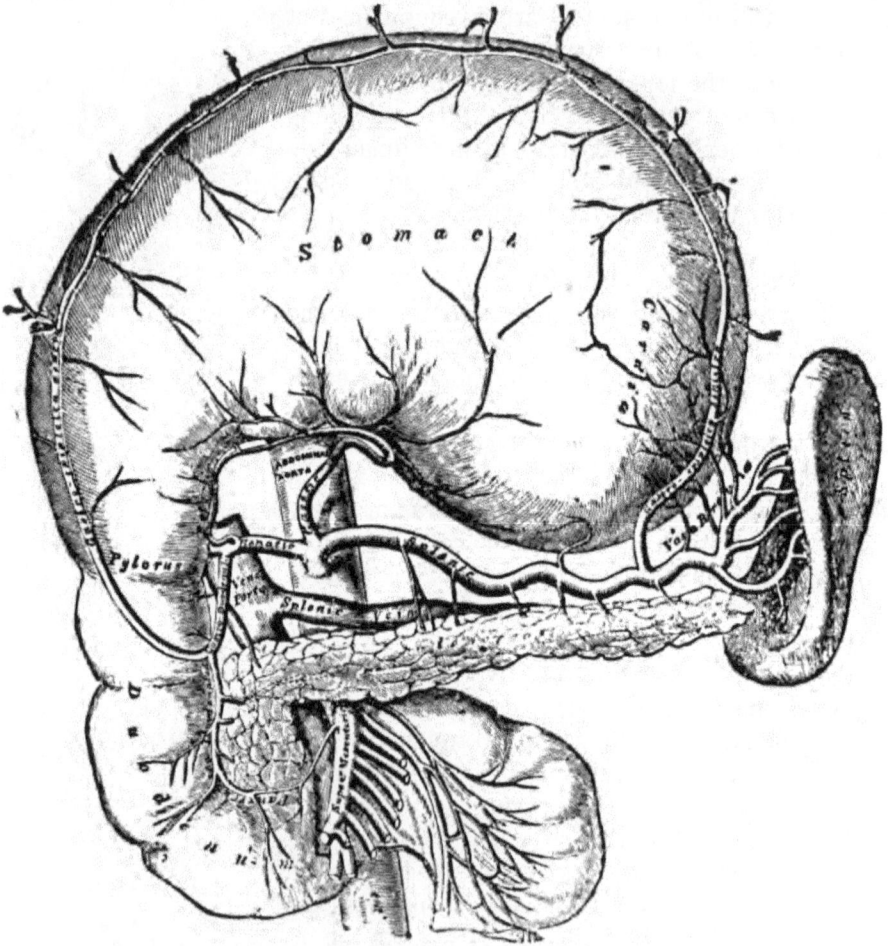

The Coeliac Axis and Its Branches, the Stomach Having Been Raised

A. Describe the coeliac axis.

A. The coeliac axis arises just below the diaphragm, comes forward half an inch and divides into the gastric, hepatic and splenic arteries, occasionally giving off one of the phrenics.

Q. Describe the gastric artery.

A. The gastric artery is one of the divisions of the coeliac axis, and supplies the stomach along its lesser curvature, anastomosing with the aortic, oesophageal, splenic and hepatic branches.

Q. Describe the hepatic artery.

A. The hepatic artery, also a division of the coeliac axis, supplies the liver and divides in the transverse fissure into many branches, supplying the different lobes of that organ.

Q. Describe the splenic artery.

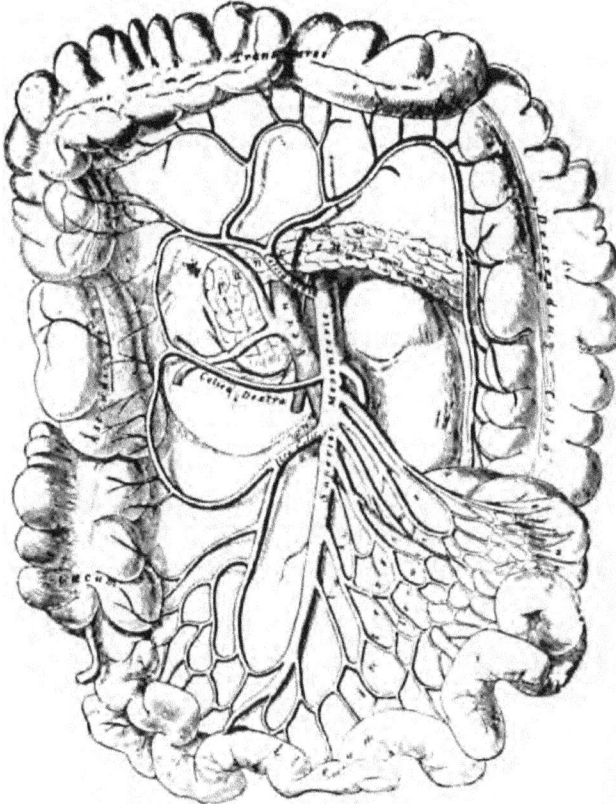

The Superior Mesenteric Artery and Its Branches

A. The splenic artery supplies the spleen and a part of the stomach, and is the largest of the three divisions of the coeliac axis. Before entering the spleen this artery divides into three branches, some of which enter the spleen and supply the substance of that organ, while others are distributed to the stomach.

Q. Describe the phrenic arteries.

A. The phrenic arteries are two in number, one on either side, usually only one arising from the aorta, the other springing from either the coeliac axis or the renal artery. They pass to the under surface of the diaphragm.

Q. Describe the mesenteric arteries.

A. The superior mesenteric artery supplies most of the small intestines, the caecum, ascending and transverse colon. It arises about one-quarter inch below the coeliac axis and arches forwards, downwards, and to the left, giving off four branches. This vessel is of large size, having many branches which ramify over the intestines.

Q. Describe the renal arteries.

A. The renal arteries, two in number, arise one from either side of the aorta, just below the mesenteric, and pass to the kidneys, entering them at the hilum. They are very large vessels, considering the size of the organs which they supply.

Q. Describe the supra-renal arteries.

A. The supra-renal arteries arise from either side of the aorta, opposite the origin of the superior mesenteric, passing to the supra-renal capsules and supplying those organs.

Q. Describe the lumbar arteries.

A. The lumbar arteries are usually four on each side of the aorta. They each divide into two branches.

Q. Describe the common iliac arteries.

A. The common iliac arteries, the divisions of the abdominal aorta, extend from the bifurcation of that vessel at the fourth lumbar vertebra, downward and outward about two inches, where they each divide into the external and internal iliac arteries.

Q. Describe the internal iliac artery.

A. The internal iliac artery is about one and one-half inches long and descends into the pelvis, where, with its branches, it supplies the bladder in the male, the bladder and womb in the female, together with a part of the generative organs.

Q. Describe the external iliac artery.

A. The external iliac artery, a continuation of the common iliac, extends to beneath the centre of Poupart's ligament, where it enters the thigh and becomes the femoral artery.

Q. Describe the femoral artery.

A. The femoral artery, a continuation of the external iliac, commences at the termination of that vessel just behind Poupart's ligament and extends downward along the fore part and inner side of the thigh for about two-thirds its length, where it becomes the popliteal artery. The femoral artery lies in the middle of a triangular space which is known as Scarpa's triangle, the outer side of which is formed by a long muscle called sartorius, the inner side by the adductor longus, and above by Poupart's ligament.

Q. Describe the popliteal artery.

A. The popliteal artery commences at the termination of the femoral and passes obliquely downwards and outwards behind the knee joint to the popliteus muscle, where it divides into two branches, the anterior and posterior tibial arteries.

Q. Describe the anterior tibial artery.

A. The anterior tibial artery commences at the bifucation of the popliteal and extends to the front of the ankle joint, where it becomes the dorsalis pedis artery.

Q. Describe the posterior tibial artery.

A. The posterior tibial artery, the larger branch of the popliteal, commences at the bifurcation of that vessel and descends obliquely to the heel, where it divides into the external and internal plantar arteries.

Q. Describe the internal plantar artery.

A. The internal plantar artery is the smaller of the terminating branches of the posterior tibial and extends along the inner side of the foot and toe.

Q. Describe the external plantar artery.

A. The external plantar artery sweeps across the plantar aspect of the foot in a curve, the convexity of which is directed outward and forward; and at the interval between the bases of the first and second metatarsal bones it inosculates with the communicating branch from the pedis dorsal, forming the plantar arch. This artery has numerous branches.

Q. What parts are supplied by the external carotid arteries and their branches?

A. The face and scalp.

Q. What arteries supply the brain?

A. The internal carotid and vertebral.

Q. What is the circle of Willis?

A. An anastomosis at the base of the brain between the branches of the internal carotid and vertebral arteries.

Q. What is the function of the circle of Willis?

A. To equalize the cerebral circulation.

Q. What arteries supply the heart?

A. The coronary arteries.

Q. What do you mean by thoracic aorta?

A. All that part of the vessel above the diaphragm and below the third dorsal vertebra.

Upper Portion of Lower Extremity. Showing Femoral Artery and Vein

Q. Which are the most important branches of this division to the embalmer?

A. The bronchial arteries, because they convey fluid to the lungs.

Q. Which of the divisions of the coeliac axis supply the liver?

A. The hepatic.

Q. Which supply the spleen?

A. The splenic.

Q. Which supply the stomach?

A. The gastric.

O. Name the arteries arising in the heart and describe each.

A. The aorta rises from the left ventricle of the heart and through its branches and sub-branches conveys pure blood to the various organs of the body. The pulmonary arteries originate in the right ventricle of the heart and convey venous or impure blood to the lungs for purification. The coronary arteries, two in number, arise from the arch of the aorta just behind the semilunar valves and ramify through the heart, supplying its substance with nourishment. The last named arteries, while not arising in the heart, nevertheless supply that organ with pure blood and may be said to be arteries of the heart.

The Arteries of the Base of the Brain, the Right Half of the Cerebellum and Pons Removed

Q. Is the right common carotid artery a continuation of the innominate or a branch?

A. It may be called a terminating branch, but it is more properly a division. It is certainly not a continuation.

Q. Name the branches of the common carotid artery?

A. The common carotid artery usually has no branches, but it occasionally gives origin to the superior thyroid, or a laryngeal branch, the inferior thyroid, and very rarely the vertebral artery. The terminating branches, or more properly speaking, the divisions of the common carotid artery are the external and internal carotid arteries.

Q. Commencing at the arch of the aorta, name the descending trunk arteries.

A. It is a question as to what constitutes a trunk artery in the mind of the formulator of this question. The principal descending trunk arteries are the thoracic and the abdominal aorta.

What may be called the minor trunk arteries are branches of the aorta: the coeliac axis, superior and inferior mesenteric, common iliac, external iliac, femoral, popliteal, and perhaps the anterior and posterior tibial.

Q. Commencing at the aorta name the trunk arteries of the right & left arm.

A. Properly speaking, the arteries of the arm do not commence at the aorta, but if they may be said to do so they are as follows: On the right side the innominate, right subclavian, axillary, brachial, and perhaps the radial and ulnar; and on the left the same, except that there is no innominate artery on that side. (The reader will observe that the arteries leading to the arm are given as well as those directly supplying that organ.)

Q. In your practice do you find exceptions or the rule to prevail in the location of arteries and veins?

A. This is rather a strange question. If the exception prevailed then the exception would become the rule. Usually both arteries and veins will be found in their normal condition, but occasionally anomalies are found.

Q. Are muscles found in the inner layer of the arteries voluntary or involuntary?

A. The muscular walls of the arteries are involuntary. Voluntary muscles are those under control of the will. Involuntary muscles those not under control of the will.

Q. Name some of the anomalies of the brachial artery.

A. The brachial artery usually bifurcates at a point half an inch below the bend of the elbow, but sometimes the bifurcation commences near the origin of the brachial artery, and the divisions continue downward as two brachial arteries instead of one. On opening the sheath the embalmer will sometimes be surprised by finding tour vessels instead of three. It makes no difference which of the arteries are used. It occasionally happens that the artery continues downward until about midway of the muscle as one single vessel, and there divides into two arteries. These divisions will continue downward until within two inches of the usual point of division, where they will join, dividing again at the usual point.

Q. Where are the most anomalous conditions found in the arteries?

A. In the brachial space.

Q. What artery arises just below the coeliac axis?

A. The superior mesenteric artery.

Q. What organs does it supply?

A. Most of the small intestine, the caecum, the ascending and transverse colon.

Q. What artery supplies the rest of the large intestines?

A. The inferior mesenteric.

Q. What arteries supply the kidneys?

A. The renal arteries.

Q. Where do they arise?

A. One from either side of the aorta; nearly opposite the origin of the superior mesenteric artery.

Q. Where is the plantar arch?

A. In the hollow of the foot.

Q. Of what artery is the superior profunda a branch?

A. Of the brachial artery.

Q. Name and locate the important arteries used in embalming.

A. They are the radial, brachial, common carotid and femoral. They have already been located.

Q. Of what is the femoral artery a branch?

A. It is not a branch; it is a continuation of the external iliac artery.

Q. Name the branches of the femoral artery.

A. Superficial epigastric, superficial circumflex iliac, superficial external pudic, deep external pudic, profunda femoris, external circumflex, internal circumflex, anastomotica magna, and the three perforating arteries.

Q. Will an embalmer run any risk of flushing the face by injecting the femoral artery?

A. Very little, if the fluid is injected very slowly, but if rapid injection is to be done the operator had best use the brachial or carotid artery.

Q. Is it necessary for the embalmer to know the names of the branches of the arteries?

A. No; a general knowledge of the arteries and their branches is all that is required; but, he who would excel in his profession cannot have too great a knowledge of the human body.

Q. Which of the arteries used in embalming do you consider the most practical and why?

A. This question must be answered by the embalmer as he thinks best. Personally, I prefer the brachial artery for ordinary use, because, first, it is very superficial throughout its entire course, and is easily secured, second, it being in the upper arm the part where the incision is made can be bandaged instead of sewed, which is a great advantage, and the mutilation cannot be seen as it can when either the radial or common carotid is used. Again, this vessel is about the right size, the radial being very small and the common carotid larger than desirable. Reasons may easily be given for preferring any of the four arteries commonly used by embalmers.

The Capillaries

Q. Describe the capillaries.

A. The capillaries are very minute blood vessels, forming a network between the terminating arteries and commencing veins. They received their name from the word capillus, a hair. They are one-thirty-five-hundredths to one-three-thousandths of an inch in diameter, and are so plentiful in the body that a cambric needle cannot be inserted in the flesh without pricking them.

The Veins

Q. What are veins?

A. Veins are tubular vessels which return the blood from the capillaries to the heart. The veins of the body may be divided as follows: Pulmonary and systemic, superficial and deep, and the sinuses.

Q. In what part of the body are the veins found?

A. They are found in all fleshy parts of the body. They have their origin in the capillaries, or rather in a minute plexus which communicates with the capillaries.

Q. How many coats have veins? Name them.

A. Like arteries they have three coats; inner, serous; middle, muscular; outer, fibrous.

Q. How do the pulmonary veins differ from all other veins in the body?

A. The pulmonary veins are distinguished from all other veins of the body by the fact that they convey pure blood from the lungs, where they originate, to the left auricle of the heart. All other veins carry impure blood.

Q. What are the systemic veins?

A. The systemic veins include all the veins of the body except the pulmonary and portal veins, the latter system being an appendage of the systemic.

Q. Describe the portal veins.

A. The portal veins are the superior and inferior mesenteric, splenic and gastric veins. They collect the blood from the digestive organs, and by their union behind the head of the pancreas form the portal vein, which enters the transverse fissure of the liver, where it divides into two branches. These, again, subdivide, ramifying throughout that organ, therein receiving blood from the branches of the hepatic artery. Its contents enter the inferior vena cava by the hepatic vein. The portal vein is about four inches long. It receives the gastric and cystic veins, and is formed by the union of the superior mesenteric and splenic veins; the inferior mesenteric joining the splenic, which also receives one of the gastric, the other emptying into the portal. These veins are often called the food veins.

Q. Describe the superficial veins.

A. The superficial veins are found between the layers of superficial fascia just beneath the skin. These veins are unaccompanied by arteries and communicate with the deep veins by branches, which pierce the deep fascia or sheath in which these vessels are contained.

Q. Describe the deep veins.

Veins of the Head and Neck

40

A. The deep veins accompany the arteries and are found in the same sheath with those vessels. The smaller arteries, as a rule, are accompanied by two veins, one on either side of the artery. They are usually known by the same name as the vessel which they accompany, but are often called venae comites, which means accompanying veins.

Q. Describe the cerebral veins.

A. The cerebral veins are remarkable for their absence of valves and for their extremely thin coat. The superficial cerebral veins are situated on the surface of the hemispheres of the brain, lying in the grooves of the convolutions. They are named from the positions they occupy upon the surface of this organ, either superior or inferior, internal or external, anterior or posterior. They originate in the capillaries and terminate in the sinuses of the dura mater.

Q. Describe the internal jugular vein.

A. The internal jugular vein receives the blood from the cranium, face and neck. It has its origin at the base of the skull and is formed by the junction of the lateral and inferior petrosal sinuses. It passes vertically, down the sides of the neck, on the outer side of the common carotid arteries, and joins the subclavian vein, forming the veins known as the venae innominatae, which unite it with the superior vena cava, the great trunk vein of the upper portion of the body.

Q. Describe the veins of the upper extremities.

A. The veins of the upper extremities are in two sets, superficial and deep. The deep follow the same course as the arteries, usually as venae comites, and have their origin in the hand, beginning as digital interosseous and palmar veins. They unite in the deep radial and ulnar, which unite at the bend of the elbow to form the accompanying veins of the brachial artery. The superficial veins lie between the layers of the superficial fascia just beneath the skin.

Q. Describe the basilic vein.

A. The basilic vein is formed by the union of the anterior and posterior ulner. It passes upward along the outer border of the triceps muscle, following the course of the brachial artery, and terminates in the axillary vein.

Q. Describe the axillary vein.

A. The axillary vein is a continuation of the basilic, and accompanies the axillary artery, terminating immediately under the clavicle, or collar bone, where it becomes the subclavian vein.

Q. Describe the subclavian vein.

A. The subclavian vein is a continuation of the axillary, which accompanies the subclavian artery until it joins with the internal jugular vein to form the innominate vein.

Q. Describe the innominate veins.

A. The innominate veins are two large trunk vessels, one on each side of the roots of the neck, and connect the internal jugular veins with the superior vena cava.

Q. Describe the superior vena cava.

A. The superior vena cava, the great trunk vein of the upper portion of the body, receives the blood from all that portion above the diaphragm. It is a short vessel about two and one-half inches in length, formed by the junction of the two innominate veins. This vein commences at the junction of the first cartilage with the sternum, and, descending, enters the pericardium above the heart and terminates in the right auricle.

Q. Describe the cardiac veins.

A. They are the great cardiac, posterior cardiac, anterior cardiac, and the venae thebesii. The function of these veins is to return the blood from the substance of the heart to the right auricle.

Q. Describe the veins of the lower extremities.

A. The veins of the lower extremities commence in the venae comites of the dorsalis pedis and plantar arteries, which unite to form the anterior and posterior tibial and peroneal veins; they collect the blood from the deep parts of the foot and leg, and unite in the popliteal, which becomes the femoral vein.

Q. Describe the femoral vein.

A. The femoral vein is a continuation of the popliteal and accompanies the femoral artery to the commencement of that vessel at Poupart's ligament. The extreme upper portion of this vessel lies posterior to the femoral artery.

Q. Describe the long saphenous vein.

A. It commences at the upper and inner side of the foot and passes upwards until it terminates in the femoral vein at about one inch below Poupart's ligament.

Q. Describe the iliac veins.

A. The iliac veins commence at the termination of the femoral just below Poupart's ligament, and accompany the iliac arteries to their termination at the commencement of the inferior vena cava.

Q. Describe the inferior vena cava,

A. The inferior vena cava is the great trunk vein of the lower portion of the body, and receives the blood from all that portion below the diaphragm. It commences at the junction of the two common iliac veins, near the fifth lumbar vertebra (fifth joint of the lumbar portion of the backbone) and passes upward on the right side of the aorta, under the liver, and piercing the diaphragm, enters the pericardium and terminates at the back and lower portions of the right auricle of the heart. This vessel has no valves other than the remains of the Eustachian valves, which are situated at the entrance to the right auricle.

Q. How do the pulmonary differ from the systemic veins?

A. The pulmonary veins convey pure blood from the capillaries of the lungs to the left auricle of the heart. The systemic veins convey impure blood from the capillaries to the right auricle of the heart.

Median Cephalic

External
Cutaneous Nerve

Internal
Cutaneous
Nerve

Median
Basilic

PECTORALIS MAJOR

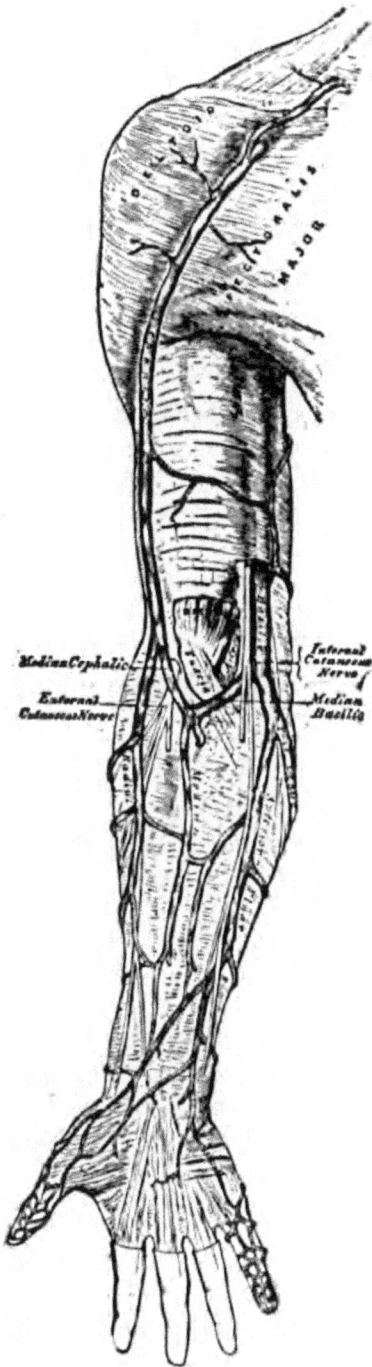

**Superficial Veins of
The Upper Extremity**

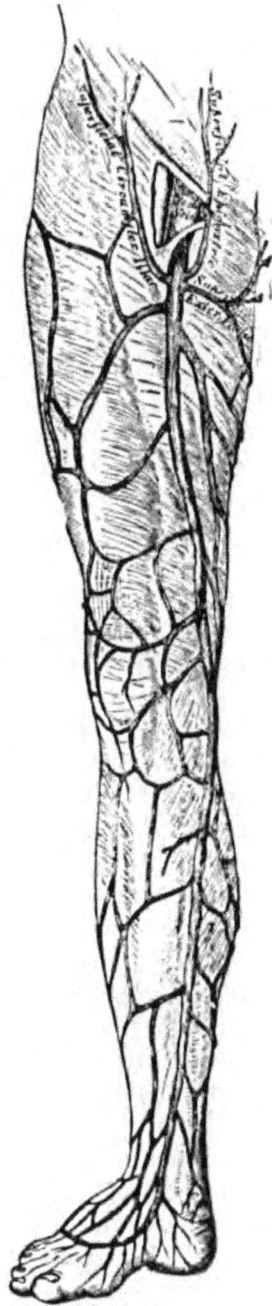

**The Long Saphenous
Vein and Branches**

Q. Name the veins of the neck which are of most importance to the embalmer.

A. The internal jugular veins.

Q. What vessels unite to form the internal jugular veins?

A. The lateral and inferior petrosal sinuses.

Q. Do veins convey blood to or from the heart?

A. All vessels conveying blood to the heart are veins; all vessels conveying blood from the heart are arteries.

Q. Are there any valves in the superior or inferior vena cava?

A. There are not.

Q. Are there any valves in the internal jugular vein?

A. There are a pair of valves near its termination.

Q. How then can the blood be forced to the face through those vessels?

A. The valves are so placed as not to hinder the passage of the blood.

Q. What veins unite to form the superior vena cava?

A. The innominate veins.

Q. What veins have no valves?

A. The cerebral, pulmonary, portal, spinal, uterine, ovarian, superior and inferior vena cava and some of the smaller veins.

Q. In what veins are most valves found?

A. In those of the lower limbs, the seat of most muscular pressure, and where the blood flows upward.

Q. Which is the longest vein in the body?

A. The internal or long saphenous vein.

Q. Give the relation of the femoral vein to the femoral artery.

A. In its upper portion it lies just at the inner side of that vessel; lower down it is found very nearly under the artery.

Q. What veins form the inferior vena cava?

A. The right and left common iliac veins.

Q. What is the use of the valves in the veins?

A. To prevent regurgitation.

Q. Are the hepatic veins a part of the portal system?

A. No; but they return the blood which has been conveyed to that organ by the portal veins from the liver to the inferior vena cava.

Q. What are those veins called which accompany the smaller arteries in pairs?

A. Venae comites.

Q. What veins unite to form the basilic vein?

A. The anterior and posterior ulnar.

Q. What are the azygos veins?

A. They connect the superior and inferior vena cava, supplying the place of those vessels in that part of the chest occupied by the heart.

Q. What veins beside the superior and inferior vena cava empty directly into the heart?

A. The pulmonary veins empty into the left auricle of the heart and the coronary sinus into the right.

Q. Commencing at the superior vena cava, name the trunk veins of the right and left arm.

A. The innominate, subclavian, axillary, basilic, cephalic, and perhaps some of the minor veins formed by the union of smaller vessels.

Q. Describe the coronary sinus.

A. It is that part of the great cardiac vein that enters into the right auricle of the heart. It is about one inch in length, is considerably dilated, and is covered by the muscular fibres of the left auricle.

Q. What are sinuses?

A. Venous channels. They perform the functions of veins and are very nearly related to those vessels. Most of them are found in the cranium. There are also grooves in the bones called sinuses.

Q. Where does the general or systemic circulation begin?

A. At the left ventricle of the heart.

Q. Where does it end?

A. At the right ventricle.

Q. How are the systemic and pulmonary circulations united or connected?

A. The pulmonary circulation begins at the right ventricle where the systemic ends, and ends at the left ventricle where the systemic begins.

Q. What trunks of the three circulations contain arterial blood?

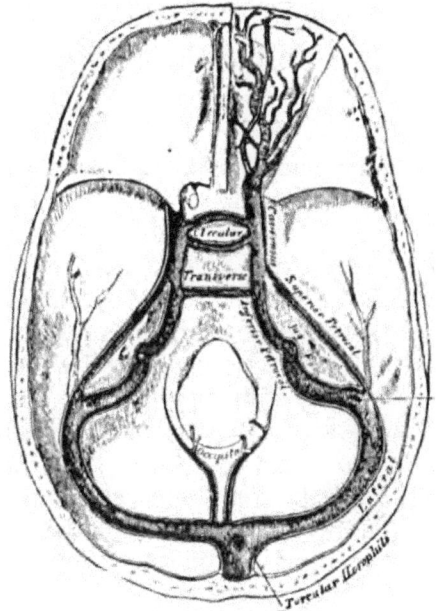

The Sinuses at the Base of the Skull

A. The pulmonary veins and the great aorta.

Q. Which ones contain venous blood?

A. The superior and inferior vena cava, the portal vein, the coronary sinus and the pulmonary artery.

Q. What veins return the blood from the spleen, kidneys, large and small intestines?

A. From the spleen the splenic vein, from the kidneys the renal veins, and from the large and small intestines the superior and inferior mesenteric veins.

Q. What veins return the blood from the lungs, heart, liver and stomach?

A. From the lungs the pulmonary and bronchial veins, from the heart the cardiac veins, from the liver the hepatic, and from the stomach the gastric.

Q. What veins return the blood from the hands and arms to the right auricle of the heart?

A. The deep veins returning the blood follow the course of the arteries in pairs and are known by the same name as the vessels they accompany, or as venae comites. The superficial veins returning the blood from the arms are the anterior ulnar, posterior ulnar, radial, median basilic, median cephalic, basilic and cephalic veins. All of these vessels, both superficial and deep, terminate in the axillary vein, which at a point near the origin of the first rib becomes the subclavian, which unites with the internal jugular vein to form the innominate. The two innominate veins unite to form the superior vena cava, which terminates in the right auricle of the heart.

Miscellaneous Questions

Q. State the difference between an artery and a vein.

A. Anatomically an artery differs from a vein in that the walls of the arteries have much more muscular tissue in their composition than veins; therefore, the walls of the arteries as compared to those of veins are very thick. Most veins have valves while arteries have none; all systemic arteries originate at the left ventricle of the heart and terminate in the capillaries, while systemic veins originate in a capillary plexus and terminate in the right auricle of the heart. Systemic arteries convey pure or oxygenated blood from the left ventricle of the heart to the capillaries, while systemic veins gather the impure blood from the capillaries and convey it to the right auricle of the heart.

Q. Name the great trunk vessels of the body and give the function of each.

A. The great trunk vessels of the body are the aorta, the superior and inferior vena cava, the portal vein, the pulmonary artery and the pulmonary veins. There are other trunk vessels, but these are the principal ones. The function of the aorta is to receive the pure blood from the left ventricle of the heart and through its branches and sub-branches distribute it to all parts of the body. The function of the superior and inferior vena cava is to receive the blood from their tributaries and convey it to the right auricle of the heart. The function of the pulmonary artery is to receive the impure blood from the right ventricle of the heart and distribute it through its divisions and subdivisions to the lungs for purification. The function of the pulmonary veins is to receive the pure blood from the capillaries of the lungs and convey it to the left auricle of the heart. The portal vein receives the blood conveyed to it by its tributaries from the organs of digestion and spleen, and conveys it to the liver.

Q. Give a description of the arteries and the office they perform in life, also of the veins.

A. A description of these vessels has already been given, but the question should be answered briefly as follows: — Arteries are tubular vessels, their function being to convey blood from both ventricles of the heart to all parts of the body, or to the capillaries. They are of two classes, systemic and pulmonary. The pulmonary arteries arise at the right ventricle of the heart and convey venous blood to the lungs for purification. The systemic arteries arise at the left ventricle of the heart, as the great aorta, which through its branches and sub-branches conveys pure or oxygenated blood to the tissues of the body for nourishment. Arteries have three coats; an inner, serous; middle, muscular, and outer, fibrous (the only coat which is vascular). Veins like arteries are also tubular vessels, their function being to convey blood from the capillaries to the auricles of the heart. There are two classes of veins, systemic and pulmonary. The pulmonary veins receive the pure blood from the capillaries of the lungs and convey it to the left auricle of the heart. The systemic veins receive the impure or carbonized blood from the capillaries and convey it to the right auricle of the heart.

Q. Which are the most important of all the blood vessels of the body?

A. The capillaries, because they bring the fluid into intimate relation with the tissues of the body.

Q. How do the capillaries nourish the tissues in life?

A. The fluid which escapes from the capillaries, known as lymph, irrigates, and nourishes the tissues.

Q. How do embalming fluids preserve the body after death?

A. The chemicals held in solution in water are absorbed by the tissues, the bacteria are destroyed, and the process of putrefaction indefinitely delayed.

Q. What is the relative capacity of the arteries and capillaries?

A. Authorities differ, giving the capacity of the capillaries as from three to eight hundred times greater than that of the arteries.

Q. Describe arteries, veins and nerves fully, stating the difference between them.

A. The difference between arteries and veins has already been described. A nerve differs from either of these vessels in that it is a bundle of fibres and when rolled between the fingers can easily be distinguished from a vessel by its firmness or solidity. In color a nerve is much the same as an empty vessel, but differs much in its general appearance.

Q. Explain the function of the lymphatics.

A. They are transparent vessels commonly called the absorbent vessels of the body. They absorb the lymph, which is thrown off by the blood, and convey it to the subclavian vein through the lymphatic and thoracic ducts.

The Blood

Q. Give the composition of the blood.

A. Water 795 in 1000 parts, corpuscles or globules 150 parts, albumen 40 parts, mineral matter 8 parts, other animal matters 5 parts, fibrine 2 parts.

Q. What are blood corpuscles?

A. Very minute, jelly-like discs in the form of a small coin. The red corpuscles are about one-thirty-two-hundredths of an inch in diameter, and about one-six-thousandths of an inch thick. White corpuscles are about one-third larger and comparatively few.

Q. What is the haemoglobin of the blood?

A. The coloring matter. When oxygen comes in contact with this substance it causes the bright red color, characteristic of the blood.

Q. What causes coagulation of the blood?

A. That constituent of the blood called fibrine, which constitutes only two-thousandths of its composition.

Q. What is the difference between arterial and venous blood?

A. Arterial blood contains oxygen and is pure; venous blood contains carbonic acid gas and is often called carbonized blood.

Q. What parts of the body contain arterial blood in life?

A. The right side of the heart, the systemic veins and the pulmonary artery.

Q. What part of the human body is blood?

A. Authorities differ, giving from one-thirteenth to one-eighth of the weight of the human body as blood; probably the last estimate is more nearly correct.

Q. What is the normal temperature of the blood?

A. It varies from 98°F. at the surface of the body to 107°F. in the hepatic vein.

Q. Where does the blood go after death?

A. Usually it leaves the arteries, most of the capillaries and superficial veins and flows into the deep veins.

Q. What causes the blood to leave the arteries?

A. By the nervous contraction of the muscular walls of the arteries, which continues after the heart ceases to force blood into the aorta; the blood in these vessels is forced into, and in most cases through, the capillary network, which is very short, to the veins; gravitation takes it from the superficial into the deep veins.

Q. What blood vessels are found empty after death?

A. The arteries and usually the pulmonary veins; however, there are exceptions to this rule.

Q. How many functions has the blood? Describe them.

A. Two; it serves to convey nutrition to the tissues and to collect those waste substances resulting from the changes constantly going on in the body, and convey them to those organs whose function it is to discharge them. It is also the medium by which oxygen is supplied to the tissues.

Q. In the process of arterial embalming, into what vessels is the blood forced?

A. What may remain in the arteries and capillaries is forced into the deep veins.

Q. Of what practical importance to the embalmer is the fact that the blood accumulates in the deep veins of the body after death?

A. It leaves the arteries and capillaries empty for injection, and it allows an easier and more convenient method of drawing blood than would be the case if it remained in all the vessels of the body.

Q. How much blood can be withdrawn from the average body after death?

A. The quantity that can be obtained varies with the size and condition of the body, and with the consistency of the blood, whether more or less coagulated. From one pint to three quarts is the average quantity; in rare cases much more. The largest quantity ever removed by the writer from one body was six quarts; this was a subject weighing two hundred and twenty-five pounds, that died suddenly of heart trouble.

Q. Do you believe it very necessary to remove blood for the perfect preservation of a dead body by embalming? If so, name three cases that require it, and three that do not require it.

A. It is seldom necessary to remove blood for the preservation of a dead body; but for cosmetic effects it is often advisable to do so. It is expedient to remove blood in septicemia, pyemia, or puerperal fever, for in these cases it contains multitudes of both pathogenic and putrefactive germs which will be removed with the blood. It is advisable to remove blood in cases of heat stroke or insolation, as in these cases the fluid is very dark, approaching to black, and should it find its way into the exposed parts of the body serious discolorations might result. It is seldom required in consumption, general senility, or anemia.

Q. If on opening an artery for injection you find that it contains blood, how would you proceed to remove it? How much would you expect to remove?

A. I would raise the femoral artery and insert as large a tube as that vessel would accommodate; to this I would attach about three feet of rubber tubing and lead the free end into an empty fluid bottle; I would then proceed to inject the artery I had previously raised and force the blood out from the femoral; when the fluid, appeared clear I would tie up the last named vessel and finish the injection. I should expect to remove from one-half to one pint of blood.

Q. When you have tied the femoral artery, is there not danger that the leg below the ligature might not receive the fluid?

A. If the ligature was placed just below the largest branch of the femoral artery, called the profunda femoris, there would be no danger of this; however, if the femoral is not tied behind the incision and there is collateral circulation the fluid will appear and flow from the cut; should it not appear, collateral circulation has not been established, and the tube must be turned and the vessel injected toward the distal end.

Q. What is the cause of blood flowing from the nostrils or mouth during arterial injection? What do you do to prevent it?

A. When clear blood flows from the mouth or nostrils it may be that blood vessels have become ruptured in the pulmonary or bronchial circulation, or possibly in the stomach during life, and there has been internal bleeding. The pressure exerted by the fluid as it passes into the body forces the blood upward as hemorrhage does in life. I have had a case in which death was caused by typhoid fever, where more than one and one-half pints of blood flowed from the nostrils. It seemed to come from the head and appeared like nose bleed in life, and it is my opinion that the blood came from the sinuses of the dura mater. The foramen caecum, an aperture formed by the frontal and what is called the crista galli of the ethmoid bone, transmits a small vein from the nose to the superior longitudinal sinus, and the posterior ethmoidal artery and vein are also indirectly connected with the sinus. The pressure of the fluid probably caused a rupture of these vessels and the hemorrhage followed.

I would never attempt to stop the flow. Place a rubber apron or bib about the neck and adjust it so the blood will flow into a vessel, then continue to inject until the hemorrhage ceases. Much more harm would come from stopping the flow than from allowing it to go on.

Q. How soon after death does the blood coagulate in the body?

A. That is a question that cannot be definitely answered. Coagulation may commence in a very few hours, and it may be delayed for several days. It partially depends upon the temperature of the blood before death. The blood may be expected to coagulate very quickly in cases where death is caused by fever.

Q. Are there any known chemicals which will liquefy coagulated blood?

A. Yes; sodium chlorides (common salt), sodium sulphates and magnesium sulphates are among the best. I have had the best results from the use of magnesium sulphates injected by the needle process or into the internal jugular vein.

Q. At what point do you puncture the heart for the purpose of withdrawing blood from the body?

A. At a point midway between the third and fourth costal cartilage, close to the breast bone and close to the fourth cartilage, holding the instrument at a slight angle to the right.

Q. How many processes do you know for drawing blood?

A. Two; by the use of a vein, or by drawing directly from the right auricle of the heart.

Q. What is post mortem staining?

A. Blood remaining in the superficial veins from which the coloring matter and oxygen has escaped, leaving it dark and staining the tissue over the course of the veins. It usually appears, if at all, the second or third day after death.

Q. In what veins is the largest quantity of blood found after death?

A. In the superior and inferior vena cava.

Q. What veins are usually empty after death?

A. The pulmonary and many of the superficial veins.

Q. Are there any embalming fluids that will bleach blood or turn it red in the dead human body?

A. No; any strong formaldehyde fluid will have a tendency to turn blood to a whitish grey if it can be made to penetrate the blood vessels, but there is no fluid that will turn partially putrefied blood to its natural color.

Q. What is your idea of drawing blood? Please tell what you know about it.

A. Blood can be drawn from the basilic, axillary, internal jugular, femoral or iliac vein, but in ordinary cases the easy, quick and tidy way to draw blood is from the right auricle of the heart direct, using an aspirator and cardiac needle.

Q. Describe your method of drawing blood from the basilic or axillary vein.

A. I seldom use the basilic vein. When I wish to draw blood from the vein in the arm I raise the artery in the axillary space. The vein lies parallel with that vessel. When I have the artery ready for injection I raise the vein and place a bridge beneath it; I then place a ligature behind the bridge on which the vessel rests, and another around the vein in front of the bridge and make an incision. When this is done insert a spiral vein tube and push it as far forward as possible, the object being to reach the right auricle; now tie the tube into the vein and attach a small rubber hose, the free end of which should lead into an empty fluid bottle; then inject the axillary artery, and the pressure of the fluid will force the blood out through the vein tube.

Q. Is this method of drawing blood always a success?

A. No; if the blood is partially coagulated it is seldom or never successful, but when the blood is in a fluid condition it is a neat and successful method of removing it.

Q. Explain how you would draw blood by the use of the internal jugular vein.

A. Make a transverse incision about three inches long, commencing just over the junction of the collar and breast bones and extending outward; cut through the skin and fat and sever the muscles from their attachments. Raise the integument and expose the sheath containing the artery and vein; carefully separate the vein from its sheath, taking care not to rupture any of its small tributaries, and when released raise it to the surface. Cut diagonally across the vein and insert a large vein tube, passing it downward to the right auricle of the heart. After adjusting the ligatures properly, attach the aspirator and the blood can be easily drawn. No doubt this is the most effective method of drawing blood ever devised.

Q. What objection, if any, can be urged against this method?

A. The principal objection is the mutilation, especially in the bodies of ladies where the friends may wish to dress the neck low. But even on the bodies of men more mutilation is necessary than will always be tolerated by the friends; besides, there is always danger of an effusion of blood during this operation, and if the friends insist on being present it is a source of great embarrassment to the embalmer.

Q. How do you prevent coagulation of the blood?

A. Introduce neutral salts, as per directions already given.

Q. What is the Shroyer method of drawing blood?

A. The so-called Shroyer method is to raise the external iliac artery and vein, place a steel tube in the vein to which is attached a rubber hose, the free end of which is led into an empty fluid bottle. A tube is then placed in the artery and that vessel injected and the blood allowed to escape from the vein. Practically this same method was taught by the writer more than ten years ago, the only difference being that Mr. Shroyer makes his incision above Poupart's ligament and uses a steel tube, while I taught my students to make the incision below the ligament and to use a flexible tube.

Q. What objection can be urged against this method of drawing blood?

A. It is open to the same objections that apply to thie use of the internal jugular vein, with the additional objection that a very large quantity of fluid must be injected in order to force the blood out of the vessel, which is not only an unnecessary expense but is liable to leave the features drawn and of an ashy hue, which is anything but desirable.

Q. Are there any cases on which you would consider it expedient to use this method?

A. Yes, on a case of anasarca or tissue dropsy, if the conditions were favorable its use would be advisable.

Q. Where is the blood during life?

A. In the heart, arteries, capillaries and veins.

Q. If you open a vein to withdraw blood from the heart, do you then attach a tube to the fluid bottle and inject while the catheter is in the heart, the centre of the circulatory system?

A. I sometimes inject a small quantity of fluid in this way for the purpose of sterilizing the blood in the great veins, but not for the purpose of obtaining a circulation. When this is done great care should be used, or the blood which may remain in the deep veins will be forced to the face.

Q. How much blood is forced from the heart at each pulsation?

A. About four ounces.

Q. How much each minute?

A. An amount equal to all the blood in the body.

Q. How much blood do the chambers of the heart contain?

A. From six to eight ounces.

Q. When you use the brachial artery, through what vein would you remove the blood?

A. The basilic or axillary.

Q. How do you prefer to draw blood, from a vein or from the right auricle of the heart direct?

A. As a rule from the right auricle, but there are many cases in which I would use a vein.

Q. How do you treat extravasations of blood about the face?

A. Extravasations, the escape of blood or other fluids from the proper channels or vessels, when taking place on the face or other parts of the body, may be the result of a blow, or may be caused by a disease known as purpura. In these cases the blood quickly coagulates and it is a very difficult matter to remove the discolorations. Crushed ice mixed with salt and applied as a poultice has often been recommended, and is of some value. In these cases a good bleacher used hypodermically, and cosmetics judiciously applied, is the best way of partially overcoming the difficulty. The discolorations cannot be wholly removed.

Q. What difference in the blood would you expect to find in a body dead of alcoholism?

A. The blood contains fat and probably alcoholic poisons, but there is no essential difference between its appearance in this and other cases.

Q. Why is a tube necessary in drawing blood from the veins?

A. For convenience and cleanliness. Blood is usually removed with an aspirator, and for obvious reasons a vein tube is indispensable.

Q. In using a catheter to aspirate blood, what vessels do you raise and what organs of the body do you enter?

A. I raise the basilic, axillary, internal jugular, femoral or iliac veins. When using either the basilic, axillary or internal jugular vein I try to enter the right auricle of the heart. When using the femoral or iliac vein I enter the inferior vena cava.

Q. How much blood would you expect to remove in this way?

A. From one-half pint to four quarts.

Q. How many varieties of blood supply exist in the lungs?

A. Two; the pulmonary and the bronchial artery supply.

Q. What is the function of these two varieties?

A. The pulmonary artery supplies blood for purification. The bronchial arteries supply pure blood for the nourishment of lung tissue.

Q. How is the venous blood brought to the vesicle and exposed to the air?

A. The small branches of the pulmonary artery divide and subdivide and do not anastomose with one another. The fine capillaries are between the air vesicles, their thin wall permitting the free interchange of gases.

Q. At what speed does the blood circulate?

A. About thirty-five feet per second. The length of each pulse wave is about nine and one-half feet. When the last part of the pulse wave has passed the arch of the aorta, the first part has just reached the arterioles.

Q. What is the color of the blood in the different parts of the circulatory system?

A. In the pulmonary veins, left side of the heart and the systemic arteries, the color is scarlet, while in the systemic veins, right side of the heart and the pulmonary arteries it is a dark blue.

Q. What is the cause of these changes?

A. The oxygen of the air enters into chemical composition with the coloring matter of the blood (haemoglobin) and produces the scarlet color. On its passage through the capillaries the oxygen is given up to the tissues and the carbon-di-oxide is taken up, the loss of oxygen causing the corpuscles to lose their scarlet color.

Q. How soon after death does the blood coagulate in the body? What causes coagulation?

A. Physiologists say from ten to twenty-four hours, but experience has taught me that it is liable to coagulate in three hours and may remain in a liquid condition for several days.

The cause is that constituent of the blood called fibrine.

Q. What conditions may hinder or delay coagulation?

A. It is delayed by sodium chloride in the injected fluid, and may be delayed indefinitely by the injection of magnesium sulphates in solution, or there may be very little fibrine in the blood, in which case it will remain liquid for an indefinite period. Moderately cold weather retards the progress of coagulation.

Q. How many circulations in the body?

A. If what is called the capillary circulation, which is only a part of the systemic, be counted, there are four: systemic, pulmonary, portal (an appendage of the systemic), and the capillary. The foetal circulation is that which takes place between the mother and the unborn child.

Q. Give the systemic circulation.

A. The systemic circulation is that which takes place between the left and right ventricles of the heart, and is as follows: The pure blood is forced from the left ventricle of the heart through the semilunar valves into the great aorta, from which it is distributed through its branches and subbranches to the capillaries; after passing through these little vessels it is gathered up by the veins and conveyed to the right auricle of the heart; from the right auricle it passes through the tri-cuspid valves into the right ventricle, thus completing the systemic circulation.

Q. Give the capillary circulation.

A. It is that circulation which takes place between the arteries and veins, through the fine network of vessels, called capillaries. It is while the blood is passing through these very minute vessels that the lymph is thrown into the tissues to nourish them.

Q. Give the pulmonary circulation.

A. The pulmonary circulation commences at the right ventricle of the heart, the venous blood being forced through the semilunar pulmonary valves into the pulmonary arteries, and along those vessels to the lungs, where it is purified by oxygen; it then returns through the four pulmonary veins to the left auricle of the heart, completing the pulmonary circulation.

Q. Give the portal circulation.

A. The portal circulation is that which takes place between the food veins and the liver; the mesenteric, gastric and splenic veins unite behind the head of the pancreas to form the portal vein, which enters the liver and ramifies throughout the substance of that organ, dividing into capillaries and radicals, which again unite to form the hepatic veins, which return the blood to the inferior vena cava.

Q. Is a knowledge of the foetal circulation necessary to embalmers?

A. Not strictly necessary, but it will add to his fund of knowledge to be acquainted with it.

Q. Give the foetal circulation.

A. The foetal circulation is that which takes place between what is known as the placenta (after-birth) and the unborn child, through the umbilical cord, which is composed of two arteries and one vein, twisted around each other until they have the appearance of a cord, hence the name. The pure blood is conveyed from the placenta by the umbilical vein, which first enters the liver of the foetus, where it divides into several branches and is distributed to different parts of that organ; then through another large branch it is conveyed to the inferior vena cava and thence to the right auricle of the heart; from the right auricle it passes through what is known as the foramen ovale into the left auricle; from the left auricle it passes through the mitral valves into the left ventricle, and from the left ventricle into the aorta, whence it is distributed by means of the subclavian and carotid arteries to the head and upper extremities; from these parts the impure blood is returned by the superior vena cava to the right auricle, whence it passes to the right ventricle, and from the right ventricle into the pulmonary artery. In the adult circulation the blood would now be carried to the lungs for purification, but in the foetus the lungs are solid, or very nearly so, therefore only a very small quantity of the blood passes into them. The greater portion passes into the descending aorta, through what is known as the ductus arteriosus. From the aorta a small quantity is distributed to the lower extremities, but by far the greater portion is conveyed by the internal iliacs and their branches to the arteries of the umbilical cord, through which it is returned to the placenta, where, after receiving oxygen and salts necessary for the growth and development of the child, it returns to it again by means of the umbilical veins.

Q. Trace a blood corpuscle from the walls of the stomach to the hand and back to the right auricle of the heart.

A. The corpuscle leaves the wall of the stomach and passes through the gastric to the portal vein, and through this vessel to the liver, where it is taken up by the hepatic vein and conveyed to the inferior vena cava; through the inferior vena cava it passes to the right auricle of the heart, from the right auricle through the tri-cuspid valve, to the right ventricle, from the right ventricle through the semilunar valve, and along the pulmonary arteries to the lungs. It receives oxygen on its passage through the Capillaries of the lungs and is taken up by the pulmonary veins and conveyed to the left auricle of the heart; from the left auricle it passes through the bi-cuspid or mitral valve into the left ventricle. From this chamber of the heart it passes upwards through the semilunar aortic valves into the ascending arch of the aorta; taking its course on the right side, it then passes through the innominate artery to the subclavian, from the subclavian to the axillary and from that vessel into the brachial; from the brachial it passes through either the ulnar or radial artery to tht palmar arch, thence into the interosseous arteries, and thence to the arterioles and into the capillaries. From the capillaries it is taken up by the interosseous veins and conveyed to the radial or ulnar veins. It is then taken through those vessels to the brachial veins, from the brachial veins into the axillary, and from that vessel to the subclavian, thence into the right innominate vein, and to the superior vena cava, which conveys it to the right auricle of the heart.

Q. What is the strong putrefactive agent in the blood?

A. Both putrefactive and fermentative agents are germs. There is much more danger from fermentation than from putrefaction of the blood, as gas is a product of the germs of fermentation and the blood may be forced to the neck or face, swelling and discoloring those parts.

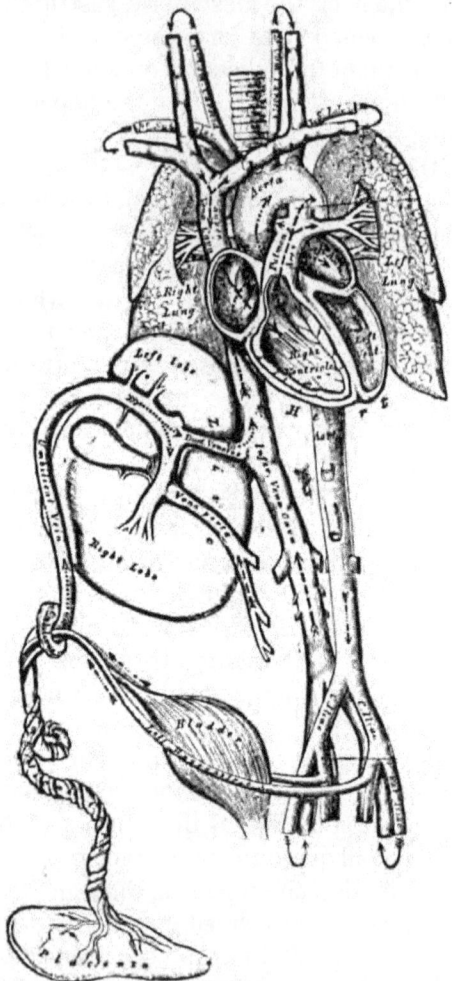

The Foetal Circulation

The Nervous System

Q. Is the nervous system of interest to embalmers?

A. With the exception of the median and ulnar nerves which serve as guides to the brachial artery and basilic vein they are of no practical interest, except such as every intelligent man should have in the entire construction of the human body.

Q. Describe briefly the nervous system.

A. The nerves originate in the brain and spinal cord, arise in pairs and by their division and sub-division are distributed over the whole body; there are forty pairs in all. Nine pairs arise from the base of the brain within the skull, and a tenth from the brain as it passes from the foramen magnum into the spine, and the remaining thirty from the spinal cord. All those nerves arising from the brain pass through the opening at the base of the skull and are distributed to the head and to those organs contained in the cavities of the thorax and abdomen. Those which arise from the spinal cord are distributed to the internal organs, the external parts of the body and to the limbs.

Q. What is the spinal cord?

A. It is a continuation of the third division of the brain, called the medula oblongata, it passes out of the head through the great opening at the base of the skull and extends downward through the canal of the backbone to the pelvis, throwing off thirty pairs of nerves in its course. At its termination it separates into almost innumerable threadlike nerves, which are sometimes spoken of collectively as the horse's tail.

Section II - The Essentials of Sanitary Science

Bacteriology

Q. What is bacteriology?

A. The science of the bacteria, their structure, form and function.

Q. What are the bacteria? Where are they found?

A. Very minute vegetable organisms; a single cell. They may be seen by the microscope at almost any time or place. They are found in the air, in water, on the surface of the earth, on the leaves of the trees, on vegetables and fruit, also in and upon the human body.

Q. How are bacteria classed?

A. By their function, as healthy, pathogenic and putrefactive. By their form: — micrococci, round shaped (streptococcus, in chains; staphylococcus, in bunches, like a bunch of grapes; diplococcus, those found in pairs; tetrads in fours, and sarcina in bales) bacilli, rod-shaped; spirilla, screw shaped.

Q. What is the function of the pathogenic bacteria?

A. They poison the living body and are bdieved to be the cause of most of the contagious and infectious diseases.

Q. What is the function of the putrefactive bacteria?

A. They cause putrefaction of the tissues and a series of chemical changes which cease only when the lately organized body has been returned to its original or inorganic elements.

Q. What is necessary to the development of bacteria?

A. Heat, moisture and congenial food.

Q. How do they increase or grow?

A. By fission or division, and by developing from spores.

Q. What are the products of bacteria and what do they cause?

A. The products of the pathogenic bacteria are disease and often death; of saprophytic, putrefaction and fermentation.

Q. What kind of bacteria develop in the living body?

A. Pathogenic bacteria, which produce nearly all forms of communicable disease.

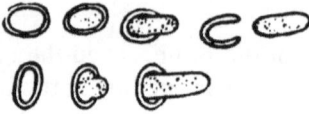

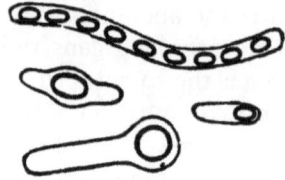

Q. What kind of bacteria develop in the dead body?

A. Saprophytic or putrefractive bacteria. They are the primary cause of putrefaction, which continues until the organic elements are changed to inorganic matter.

Q. Do saprophytic bacteria ever cause disease?

A. They do.

Q. What is a spore?

A. An undeveloped germ. The equivalent of the bud or germ cell.

Q. Describe the production of spores.

A. According to Brefield and others the process is as follows: By the absorption of water they become swollen and pale, losing their shining, refractive appearance. Later a little protuberance is seen upon one side or at one extremity of the spore, and this rapidly grows out to form a rod, which consists of soft-growing protoplasm enveloped in a membrane which is formed of the inner layer of the cellular envelope of the spore. The outer envelope is cast off and may be seen in the vicinity of the newly formed rod. Sometimes the vegetative cell emerges from one extremity of the oval spore, and in other species the exosporium is ruptured and the bacillus emerges from the side.

Q. Must special means be used for the disinfection of material believed to contain spores?

A. Yes. Spores preserve their vitality for a long time when exposed to disinfectants and are not easily destroyed by dessication. The spores of some kind of pathogenic bacteria are destroyed by boiling water in a few minutes, while others retain their vitality for half an hour or longer. In disinfection of appartments, plenty of time should be allowed, and heat and moisture used, to develop the spores, after which they are easily destroyed.

Q. Of what are the spores composed?

A. They are composed of condensed protoplasm, which retains the vital character of the soft protoplasm of the mother cell from which it has been separated.

Q. What germs form spores?

A. As far as known the following pathogenic bacteria form spores: The bacillus of anthrax, tetanus, malignant oedema, and the bacillus of symptomatic anthrax. The following as far as known do not form spores; the pus cocci, the micrococcus of pnuemonia, the bacillus of typhoid fever, the bacillus of glanders, the bacillus of diphtheria, the spirillum of cholera, the spirillum of relapsing fever.

Q. What influence has temperature on disinfection?

A. As a rule germicidal activity increases in direct proportion to the increase in temperature from 20 degrees C.

Q. What are the conditions of growth of the bacteria?

A. Bacteria only grow in presence of moisture under certain conditions and temperature and when supplied with suitable pabulum. As they do not contain chlorophyll they cannot assimilate carbon dioxide and light is not favorable to their development. The aerobic species obtain oxygen from the air and cannot grow unless supplied with it. The anaerobic species on the other hand will not grow in the presence of oxygen, and must obtain tTiis element as they do carbon and nitrogen from the organic material which serves them as food. Water is essential for the development of bacteria and many species have their normal habitat in the waters of the ocean, of lakes and of running streams, others thrive upon damp surfaces, or in the interior of moist masses of organic material." As a rule, growth is arrested when the temperature falls below 50 degrees F., but some species multiply at a still lower temperature. Low temperatures arrest the growth of bacteria, but do not destroy them.

Q. Are bacteria always present in dead bodies?

A. No better answer to this question can be given than to quote Sternburg on bacteria of cadavers. He says "The putrefactive changes which occur so promptly in cadavers when temperature conditions are favorable result chiefly from post mortem invasion of the tissues by bacteria contained in the alimentary canal. But it is probable that under certain circumstances microorganisms from the intestine may find their way into the circulation during the last hours of life, and that the very prompt putrefactive changes in certain infectious diseases in which the infection is involved is due to this fact. The writer has made numerous experiments in which a portion of the liver or kidney removed from the cadaver at an autopsy made soon after death has been enveloped in an antiseptic wrapping and kept for forty-eight hours at a temperature of from 25 to 30 degrees C. In every instance there has been an abundant development of bacteria, although as a rule none were obtained from the same material immediately after the removal of the organs from the body. This shows that a few scattered bacteria were present. The same result was obtained in case of sudden death from accident, as from portions of kidney or liver removed from the bodies of persons dying from yellow fever, tuberculosis and other diseases." This high authority would seem to prove the fact that bacteria are always present in dead bodies.

Q. What is meant by a germ?

A. A very minute vegetable organism; a single cell.

Q. What is the difference between saprophytes and parasites?

A. Saprophytes exist independent of the living body, obtaining their supply of nutriment from dead animal or vegetable material, or from water containing organic or inorganic matter in solution. The strict parasites depend upon the living body for existence, growth and multiplication. They are not always injurious to the animal on which they depend for existence, but they are sometimes very harmful, giving rise to acute and chronic diseases.

Q. State the difference between a germ and a spore.

A. A spore is a bud or germ cell, an undeveloped germ. A germ or microbe is a very minute vegetable organism, which is fully developed.

Q. What is the difference between bacteria and infusoria?

A. Bacteria are minute vegetable organisms, single cells; the lowest form of vegetable life. Infusoria is the lowest form of animal life; microscopical animals.

Q. What are bacterium?

A. An individual class of cells or germs belonging to the bacteria. By some the word bacterium is believed to mean a single cell, not a class.

Q. Are there any other forms of bacteria that can exist in either dead or living bodies?

A. Yes; there are certain micro-organisms which can exist in either living or dead tissue. They are called facultative parasites.

Q. What are chromogenic bacteria?

A. Chromogenes or chromogenic bacteria are those forms of bacterial life which form pigment or coloring matter, and those which produce fermentation, known as zymogenes, or zymogenic bacteria. These, however, according to Sternburg do not form a separate class, as many of "the species known by these names are also pathogenic.

Q. How are bacteria studied?

A. The study of bacteriology consists of investigation made by the use of a microscope, and in the artificial cultivation or culture of the germ.

Q. What is a microbe?

A. Microbe is the general name for micro-organisms or organic structures, whether they belong to what are known as bacteria, which are vegetable organisms, or the infusoria, which are animal; those organisms requiring the use of the microscope for their study.

Q. What is the difference between bacteria and microbes?

A. There is no difference, if they belong to the same family. A microbe, however, may be an animal organism, while bacteria are necessarily vegetable.

Q. How rapidly do bacteria germinate?

A. According to Sternburg, it has been demonstrated that certain bacteria will multiply at such a rapid rate that under favorable conditions one single cell may in the short space of twenty-four hours become sixteen million seven hundred and seventy-seven thousand two hundred and twenty (16,777,220).

Bacteria in Relation to Contagious Diseases

Q. Name some of the diseases which are known to be caused by the bacteria.

A. Diphtheria, typhoid fever, Asiatic cholera, erysipelas, consumption, gonorrhoea, anthrax, bubonic plague, glanders, and many others.

Q. Name the specific germ of consumption, diphtheria, typhoid fever, and Asiatic cholera.

A. Of diphtheria, dipthococcus; typhoid fever, bacillus typhosus; consumption, bacillus tuberculosis, and Asiatic cholera, common bacillus of Koch.

Q. Is scarlet fever a bacterial disease?

A. The cause of this disease is not positively known, but there is little doubt that the origin is to be found in the bacteria, although a physician of high standing and claiming to be well versed in bacteriology in speaking to the writer of the mode of communication of scarlet fever gave as his opinion that the source of infection was animal and not bacteria. However, it is certainly a highly contagious disease and one to be dreaded as it often proves fatal.

Q. Is what is known as influenza a communicable disease?

A. Influenza, or what is more popularly known by its French name, la grippe, is a highly contagious disease, and undoubtedly caused by a specific germ, the bacillus influenza. This disease received its name from the word influence, it having been at one time believed to be due to the influence of the stars. It is seldom fatal unless complicated by pneumonia; but this frequently happens and many fatalities result from what was primarily la grippe.

Q. Is typhoid fever caused by the bacteria? If so, is it contagious or infectious?

A. Yes, it is caused by a specific germ. It is not considered contagious, but infectious from infected food or drink. Raw oysters are believed to be a frequent source of the infection.

Q. What is the name of the specific germ causing this disease?

A. It is called bacillus typhosus.

Q. In what parts of the body dead of this disease are the most germs found?

A. In the interior of the bowels, in the abdominal viscera, and in the contents of the urinary bladder.

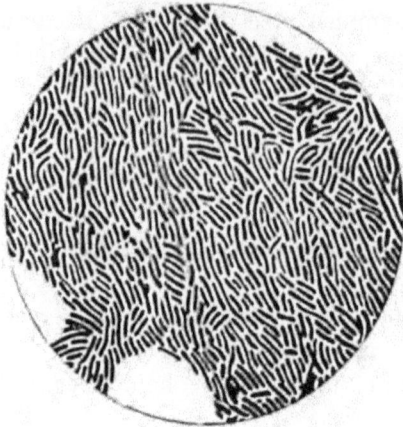

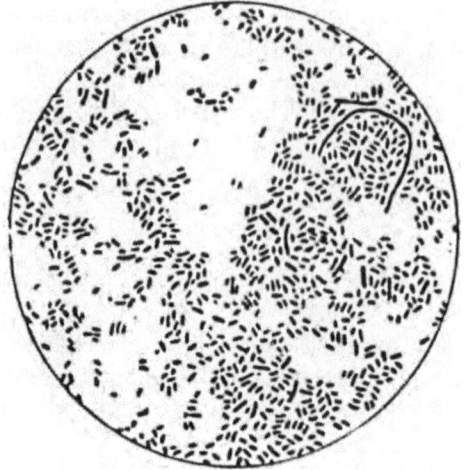

Bacillus of Typhoid Fever

Q. Is tuberculosis contagious or infectious?

A. Tuberculosis, commonly called consumption, is classed as a contagious disease, but not as one that is particularly dangerous, except to those who are constitutionally weak, or by inheritance inclined to the disease.

Q. What is the source of communication?

A. The sources of communication are almost too numerous to mention. In many cases the germs are conveyed to the alimentary canal through infected food or drink, but in by far the greater number of cases they are breathed in with the air. Undoubtedly the greatest source of contagion is the sputum deposited on the sidewalks or in the streets by people suffering from this disease. The sputum dries, the tubercle bacilli arise in the dust and are taken into the lungs, and disease and death are the result.

Q. Is yellow fever a bacterial disease?

A. It is a communicable disease, the source of which is believed to be a mosquito. It is called yellow fever on account of its tendency to turn the body yellow. It is seldom heard of in cold climates, but often visits the southern parts of the United States with very disastrous results, always subsiding and finally disappearing on the approach of cold weather. This fact is certainly a point in favor of the belief that the germ is conveyed by an insect.

Q. Is pneumonia contagious or infectious?

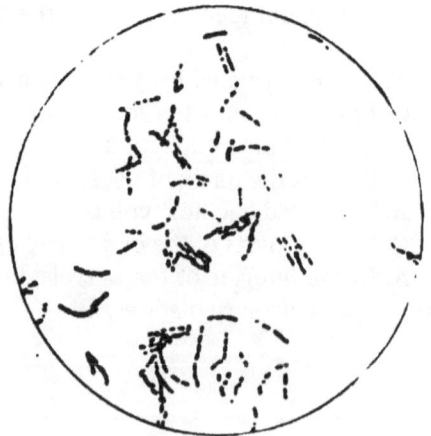

Bacillus Tuberculosis

62

A. By some it is believed to be mildly contagious, while others seriously doubt its being communicable. The fact probably is that it is communicable when the system is in the proper condition to receive the germ, and not communicable to a healthy individual. The source of infection is believed by some to be a species of bacteria, known as pneumococcus, while others think that the specific germ, if there is one, has never been discovered.

Q. Should bodies dead of this disease be disinfected before shipping?

A. They are to be considered as contagious and treated accordingly.

Q. Should the premises be disinfected after a member of the household has died of this disease?

A. Some of the Boards of Health require it and others do not. I am of the opinion that it is not necessary, provided all cloths and other material used about the patient have been burned or disinfected.

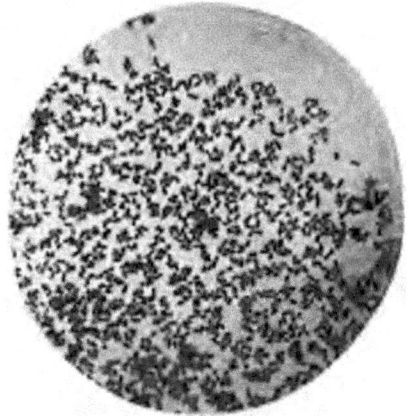

Bacillus of Diphtheria

Q. Describe the disease known as diphtheria.

A. This disease is believed to be caused by a specific germ, known as diphthococcus, but scientists are not quite certain whether it is always caused by this germ, or whether in different regions and under different conditions, it may be sometimes one and sometimes another species of germ life that causes it. It attacks the mucous membrane of the air passages, producing much depression of the vital forces, and is characterized by sore throat and membranous exudations, which usually appear on the mucous surface of the tonsils and back part of the throat. The bacillus of diphtheria can be readily destroyed by any one of the approved germicides, such as corrosive sublimate or formaldehyde.

Q. Describe smallpox. Is it contagious or infectious?

A. It is a highly contagious disease, characterized by fever and the appearance of an eruption on the surface of the body. This eruption after passing through various stages, finally dries up, leaving scars or pits on the face, commonly called pock marks.

Q. How would you disinfect such a body?

A. Usually there is an immune in charge of those sick with this disease, and if so, when death ensues he should prepare the body for burial. The body should be sponged with a strong disinfectant (1:500 bichloride of mercury is best), and then wrapped in a sheet saturated with the same disinfectant and buried as quickly as possible. Should the embalmer be obliged to do the work, he should use every precaution to prevent spreading the disease, and in time of smallpox epidemic should, of course, keep himself constantly vaccinated, which will give him immunity in ninety-five cases out of one hundred, and should he become infected, cause the disease to be of very light form.

Q. Is leprosy a contagious or an infectious disease? How would you treat a case of this kind?

A. The best authorities class this disease among those that are infectious only, while others claim that it is contagious. It is certainly communicable, but as the disease is very rarely seen in this country, it is not particularly interesting to the embalmer. Should an embalmer have a case of this kind, he should treat it as he would a syphilitic case. Disinfect the body and everything that has come in contact with it, and in order to protect himself against infection, wear rubber gloves while operating.

Q. Is syphilis contagious or infectious? What precaution should be taken in caring for a case of this kind?

A. As contagious and infectious diseases are classed and described, this is an infectious disease, as it can be taken only by inoculation. In its advanced stages putrid sores often appear on the inside of the ankles, and their syphilitic origin is easily detected by a peculiar odor. Syphilis is often an inherited disease. The biblical saying that "the iniquities of the fathers are visited upon the children even unto the third and fourth generation," whether it be considered as a threat or as a warning, is certainly as true as anything that appears in holy writ.

The embalmer cannot be too careful in handling bodies that come into his care, for he may become inoculated with the virus if there are any abrasions of the skin of the hands. He should remember that this disease is not confined to any class of society; those moving in the highest walks of life are often afflicted with it. If the disease is suspected, he should wear gloves while operating; then, should he come in contact with sores on the body, he will be safe. A case of this kind can be disinfected the same as any other contagious or infectious disease.

Q. Is there danger to the embalmer from bodies dead of typhoid fever?

A. There may be danger if he inhales the gas that may escape after puncturing the stomach or bowels, but this he should never do.

Q. What precaution should be taken in order to avoid danger of infection?

A. If the gas is to be relieved, attach a piece of rubber tubing about three feet long to the trocar, and lead the free end into a bottle of good disinfecting fluid, so that the gas can escape into it, or lead the tube out through the window, Any way to avoid breathing the gas, which may or may not be infectious, is to be recommended.

Q. What do you do with the water with which you have washed the body of one dead of typhoid fever? Is it infectious?

A. Disinfect and throw it into the sewer. It may be infectious.

Q. Is typhoid fever contagious? How is it communicable from person to person?

A. No. It is infectious and is communicable by drinking infected water or by eating infected food.

Q. After the health authorities have posted a card on a house bearing the words typhoid fever, why do they, in case death results, after taking the precaution of warning the public of the disease, allow a public funeral?

A. If it is true that tyhpoid fever can only be taken through eating or drinking infected food or water, there is no need of either the notice or a private funeral. When either or both are ordered by the health authorities, the natural conclusion would be that they are inclined to believe the disease contagious.

Q. What diseases are most dangerous to the embalmer while doing his work?

A. From inoculation, syphilis, puerperal fever, septicemia, pyemia, and gangrene. From contagion, smallpox, scarlet fever and diphtheria. There is more or less danger from the blood of any body recently dead.

Q. What precaution would you take to prevent spreading the germs in preparing a body dead of a contagious disease for burial?

A. I would provide myself with an antiseptic suit if possible; not having one, I would wear a cast-off suit of clothes, and over that a long tight fitting rubber or mackintosh coat; rubber boots should be worn on the feet, and a snug fitting silk cap on the head, completely protecting the hair. No unnecessary paraphernalia should be used or carried. When the work is done, the outside coat and clothes should be disinfected by dipping a brush in an antiseptic solution, and brushing them thoroughly. A solution of corrosive sublimate, one-half dram to two quarts of water, is the best solution for this purpose. Then take a ride in the open air before going home or to any other house. When at home, remove the clothes, place in a closet, and disinfect by spraying with formaldehyde, or by hanging cloths or sheets in the closet and spraying the formaldehyde on them; whichever is done, close the door and leave the clothes there until again wanted.

Q. How would you prepare a body dead of diphtheria for shipment to another State?

A. Sponge it thoroughly with an approved disinfectant, and be very particular about washing out the throat and nostrils, also with an approved disinfectant. I would then pack all orifices of the body with cotton, embalm arterially and fill the cavities, using a standard fluid. Then bandage the body and observe the state laws and rules of the Board of Health in regard to shipping.

Q. How would you embalm a body for burial after death from tuberculosis of the lungs?

A. Inject it arterially, fill the cavities, inject the air cells of the lungs through the trachea and see that no serous fluids remain in the body, always using a fluid known to be a disinfectant.

Q. How would you prepare a non-contagious body, that cannot reach its destination within thirty hours, for shipment?

A. Many of the Boards of Health require it to be treated as a contagious case, but I cannot see the necessity of this rule. If the body is properly embalmed there is not the slightest danger to the public health in thirty or even fifty hours.

Q. How do micro-organisms multiply or thrive?

A. With heat, moisture and congenial food.

Q. What is the relation of temperature to putrefaction?

A. It will not take place at a temperature below 32°F. Bacteria develop rapidly and cause putrefaction at a temperature ranging from 65° to 100°F.

Q. What is the relation of temperature to fermentation?

A. The same as to putrefaction.

Q. What organs are affected in case of typhoid fever?

A. The alimentary tract, liver, spleen and kidneys, and sometimes other organs.

Q. How would you prepare for burial a body dead of diphtheria?

A. Disinfect it, as instructed in other contagious cases, taking care to look after the mouth, throat and nostrils, where the greatest number of germs are to be found.

Q. What disinfection of premises, of clothing, and of yourself is necessary?

A. The same as in any highly contagious case.

Q. How would you prepare for shipment a body dead from measles?

A. Treat it as a contagious case; the directions have already been given.

Q. How would you prepare for shipment a body dead of smallpox?

A. If I am not mistaken, Michigan is the only state in the Union that would allow the case to be shipped, and that only when prepared by a licensed embalmer acting under the instructions of the Board of Health.

Q. State which is the more dangerous, an infectious or a contagious disease.

A. A contagious disease.

Q. What temperature is necessary to destroy bacteria?

A. 212 to 250 degrees F.

Q. What parts of the body contain the most germs in each of the following diseases: — tuberculosis, typhoid fever, scarlet fever and diphtheria?

A. In tuberculosis, the lungs, throat, mouth and nostrils; in typhoid fever, the interior of the bowels and other abdominal viscera; in scarlet fever, the skin, between the cuticle and derma; in diphtheria, the mouth, throat and nostrils.

Q. How are diphtheria and scarlet fever communicable?

A. As the germs are spread by atmospheric diffusion, either of these diseases may be contracted by breathing, the germs entering the respiratory tract or into the alimentary canal. Scarlet fever, like most contagious diseases, is usually contracted by breathing in the germs, but may be taken into the body with infected food. Diphtheria may be contracted in the same way.

Q. Why do health boards in many states require bodies dead of certain bacterial diseases to be wrapped in a sheet saturated with a solution of bichloride of mercury?

A. As an additional precaution and safeguard for the public. However, if all the other rules and regulations have been faithfully followed this one would seem unnecessary.

Q. How is tuberculosis usually communicated?

A. By kissing, by the sputum being allowed to dry and the germs to escape into the atmosphere, and by constant association with those afflicted with the disease.

Q. Should a house be disinfected after death has occurred from consumption?

A. It certainly should be, together with all its contents.

Q. When taking a bath to disinfect your body after attending a contagious case, what would you use in the water?

A. Bichloride of mercury; 1:2000, or one-half drachm to a gallon of water.

Q. How would you treat a case of scarlet fever?

A. In this, as in all highly contagious and dangerous cases, the work of disinfecting the body should be done in a thorough manner. The body should be thoroughly sponged with a solution of bichloride of mercury, and all orifices disinfected and packed with cotton; it should then be arterially embalmed, and all serous cavities filled with an embalming fluid known to be a disinfectant. Particular attention in this case should be given to the skin, as the most germs are believed to be beneath the cuticle. If the blood is withdrawn, it should be thoroughly disinfected before being disposed of, and underclothing, towels, etc., that have been about the patient or around the room should be put to soak in an antiseptic solution, and afterwards boiled for at least thirty minutes. Not only the room where the patient was confined, but all rooms near it, especially those frequented by the nurse and others who spent any time with the patient should be disinfected. If the body is to be shipped, it must be treated strictly in accordance with the rules of the health authorities.

Q. Is Asiatic cholera contagious or infectious? How would you treat the disease?

A. Infectious; caused by a little curved bacillus, which finds lodgement in the alimentary canal. The writer when a boy passed through an epidemic of cholera, and hopes never to see another. It seldom visits these shores, but whenever it has done so has proven very fatal.

The treatment of a cholera case should not differ materially from that of any highly infectious case. First spray the room, then sponge the body, using a good disinfecting fluid; then if the body is to be held, embalm arterially, and never fail to puncture and inject the bowels, and wash out and pack all orifices of the body. The probabilities are that the health authorities would order the body wrapped in a sheet saturated with a solution of bichloride of mercury and buried at once.

Q. What is the source of contagion in smallpox and measles?

A. The source of danger in smallpox and probably in measles is the eruptions on the surface of the body.

Q. Which is the best way to disinfect a room and its contents in order to insure the destruction of the bacteria when using sulphur, by using it dry or with moisture?

A. With moisture, as it has a tendency to develop the germs, rendering them much easier to destroy.

Q. What is meant by the word hygiene?

A. The science of the laws that promote and preserve health.

Q. What is a sanitarian?

A. One versed in sanitary science.

Q. Is the destruction of the bacteria a part of the work of a sanitarian?

A. It is.

Q. State in detail what would be the difference in your treatment of a contagious case and that of a non-contagious one, and why.

A. In a contagious case in addition to the ordinary work of embalming the body, I would be careful to use a fluid I knew to be a reliable disinfectant and a larger quantity than would be strictly necessary to preserve the body. I would then sponge the body thoroughly with an approved disinfectant, and wash and pack the apertures. I would do this in order to prevent contagion.

Q. What recommendations have been made by authorities for the prevention of the spread of diphtheria?

A. The following communications on the measures to be taken for prevention of the spread of diphtheria were made by Lofler in 1890:

The cause of diphtheria is the diphtheria bacillus which is found in the secretions of the affected mucous membrane. With this secretion it is distributed outside of the body and may be deposited upon anything in the vicinity of the sick. Those sick with diphtheria carry about bacilli capable of infecting others so long as there is the slightest trace of diphtheretic deposit, and even for several days after such deposits have disappeared.

Those sick with diphtheria are to be rigidly isolated so long as the diphtheria bacilli are present in their secretions. Children who have been sick with diphtheria should be kept from school for at least four weeks.

The diphtheria bacilli may preserve vitality in dried fragments of diphther-

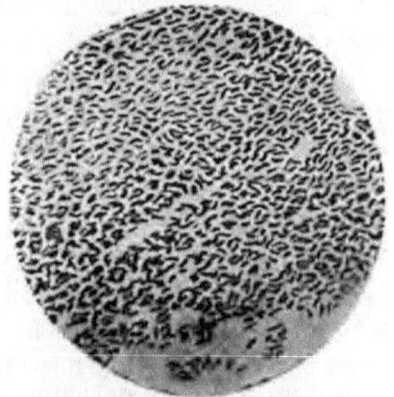

Spirillum of Asiatic Cholera

etic membrane for four or five months. Therefore, all objects which may have been exposed to contact with the excretions of those sick with diphtheria, such as linen, bed-clothing, utensils, clothing of nurses, etc., should be disinfected by boiling in water or treated with steam at 100 degrees C. In the same way the rooms occupied by diphtheria patients are to be carefully disinfected. The floors should be repeatedly scrubbed with hot sublimate solution (1:1000) and the walls rubbed down with bread.

Q. Would this recommendation apply to almost any highly contagious disease?

A. Yes.

Q. Describe separately and fully how the following diseases are communicated: Asiatic cholera, bubonic plague, diphtheria, measles, pneumonia, scarlet fever, smallpox, and yellow fever.

A. Asiatic cholera is an infectious, contagious disease which may be communicated in much the same way as typhoid fever, either by drinking infected water or milk, or by eating infected food, and many well-informed sanitarians believe that the germs are spread by atmospheric diffusion; however, others deny it. Bubonic plague may

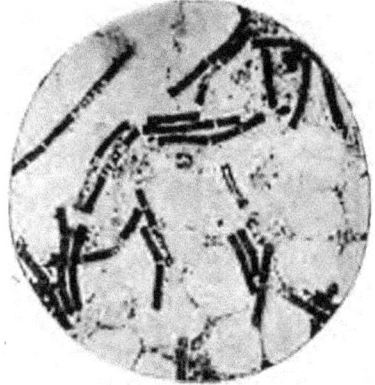

Anthrax Bacillus

be communicated through a cut, or wound, and may be spread by atmospheric diffusion, but authorities differ as to the mode of communication. Diphtheria may be communicated from the sick to the well either by contact or through the atmosphere. It is highly contagious. All material used around the body, sick or dead of this disease, should immediately be burned or disinfected. Measles is a highly contagious disease communicated through the atmosphere, but the pacific germ that causes it, if it is one, is not known. Pneumonia is believed to be a contagious disease probably communicated through the atmosphere to a person in the right physical condition to receive it. The source of the germ is probably the sputum. The source of communication in scarlet fever is not certainly known, but it is undoubtedly a bacterial disease, communicated by direct contact or by atmospheric diffusion. The germ of smallpox is not known, but it is highly contagious at any stage of the disease, or from contact with any part of the body, and the contagion is doubtless spread by atmospheric diffusion.

Disinfection and Disinfectants

Q. What is meant by disinfection?

A. The destruction of micro organisms. By some the word is also considered to mean the destruction of disagreeable odors, but this is erroneous.

Q. What is a disinfectant?

A. Any drug, chemical, or other agent capable of destroying germ life.

Q. What is an antiseptic?

A. Anything which will restrain the growth and multiplication of germs.

O. What is a deodorizer?

A. A chemical capable of destroying bad odors.

Q. Is a deodorizer necessarily an antiseptic?

A. I cannot say that I know of any good deodorizers that are not more or less of an antiseptic nature.

Q. Are deodorizers necessarily disinfectants?

A. No; very few of the chemicals used as deodorizers are reliable disinfectants.

Q. Name a deodorizer that is a disinfectant.

A. Chloride of lime; six ounces to one gallon of water.

Q. What is meant by an approved disinfectant?

A. A drug, chemical or combination of chemicals having the approval of health authorities.

Q. Name three approved disinfectants.

A. Formaldehyde, bichloride of mercury and carbolic acid.

Q. What action on bacteria has the preparation known as tri-kresol?

A. It has about the same action as carbolic acid, but it is said to be more efficient and less poisonous. One per cent in solution is said to be a good antiseptic, and three per cent a reliable disinfectant.

Q. What is lysol and of what value is it as a disinfectant?

A. A proprietary preparation believed to contain fifty per cent of kresols. It is said to possess the same disinfecting qualities as crude carbolic acid and to be less poisonous.

Q. What antiseptic powers has alcohol?

A. It is a very weak antiseptic, but owing to dehydrating qualities it is considered of value in preparing the way for stronger disinfectants.

Q. What is the best disinfectant for the excretions of the bowels in typhoid fever cases?

A. Chloride of lime in the proportion of six ounces to one gallon of water. One quart of this solution should be used for each discharge.

Q. Are there any other diseases with which you are acquainted .in which the excreta need to be disinfected?

A. Yes, dysentery, tuberculosis and diphtheria are diseases in which the excretions of the bowels should be disinfected.

Q. Will the chloride of lime solution given above destroy the germs of these diseases as well as those of typhoid fever?

A. Yes.

Q. Are there any other diseases in which the excretions of the bowels are believed to be dangerous?

A. In Asiatic cholera, and in yellow, scarlet and typhus fevers all excreta are believed to be dangerous.

Q. What value has chlorine gas as a disinfectant?

A. It is believed to be a good disinfectant and previous to the advent of formaldehyde was quite extensively used for disinfecting apartments or rooms, but is little used at the present time on account of its bleaching and oxidizing qualities.

Q. Of what value is sulphurous acid gas?

A. As a disinfectant for rooms and apartments it is believed, to be a safe disinfectant if used in the proper manner and quantity. tJut is ooen to the octmc objections as chlorine gas.

Q. What is the best gaseous disinfectant known to science?

A. Formaldehyde gas.

Q. What disinfecting powers have essential oils?

A. Experiments have been made by eminent authorities and the following table gives the essences which kill the bacillus of typhoid fever after a contact of less than twenty-four hours:

Cinnamon of Ceylon	12 minutes.	Geranium of France	50 "
Cloves	25 "	Origanum	75 "
Eugenol	30 "	Patchouly	80 "
Thyme	35 "	Zedoary	2 hours.
Wild thyme	35 "	Absinthe	4 "
Verbena of India	45 "	Sandalwood	12 "

Q. State the germicidal powers of some of the various acids.

A. Sternburg gives the experiments of himself and others with various acids. He says that in his experiments micrococci were destroyed in two hours in a 1:2000 by weight solution of sulphur dioxide added to water, and cites authority to prove that a solution of .28 per cent killed the typhoid bacillus, and of .148 per cent the cholera spirillum. The same writer says that pus cocci failed to grow in a culture solution containing one part of sulphur dioxide in five thousand of water. A five-per-cent solution of nitric acid failed to sterilize broken-down beef tea, but it was thoroughly sterilized by an eight-per-cent solution. Hydrochloric acid is a very powerful disinfectant, destroying in two hours the bacillus of typhoid fever in solution of 1:300, and the bacillus of diphtheria in 1:700, and glanders bacillus in 1:200. Chromic acid destroys anthrax spores in from one to two days in a one-per-cent solution, and prevents the development of putrefactive bacteria in solution of 1:5000. A one-per-cent solution of osmic acid kills anthrax spores in twenty-four hours. A three-per-cent solution of phosphoric acid destroys typhoid fever germs in four hours.

Acetic acid failed to kill anthrax spores after five days' exposure, but micrococci were killed in two hours by a one-percent solution. Lactic acid killed the bacillus of typhoid fever in five hours in solution of .4 per cent. Citric acid killed the germs of cholera in half an hour in solution of 1:200, and destroyed the germs of typhoid fever in five hours at .43 per cent. Oxalic acid destroyed the germs of typhoid fever in solution of .36 per cent, in five hours, and the germs of Asiatic cholera in the same length of time in solution of .28 per cent. Boracic acid is a weak disinfectant. A five-per-cent solution failed to destroy anthrax spores in five days, and a saturated solution failed to destroy pus cocci in two hours. However, it is antiseptic in a solution as weak as 1:143. Salicylic acid in two-per-cent solution destroys pus cocci in two hours. Micrococci are destroyed in solutions of 1-400. Formic acid destroys typhoid germs in five hours in solution of .35 per cent. Arsenious acid prevents putrefactive changes in solution of 1:166.

Q. What value have alkalies as disinfectants?

A. Sternburg says that in two hours a ten-per-cent solution of caustic potash was fatal to pus cocci, and an eight-percent solution failed. A ten-per-cent solution failed to destroy tuberculosis germs in twenty-four hours, while the anthrax germs were destroyed by a solution of one per cent. According to Jager soda has about the same germicidal powers as caustic potash. It acts as an antiseptic in proportion of 1:56.

Q. What germicidal powers has ammonia?

A. Experiments made by authorities prove that the typhoid bacillus were destroyed in five hours by a three-percent solution, and the germs of cholera by a solution of about the same strength. Boer says that anthrax bacillus were destroyed in two hours with a solution of 1:300. The bacillus of diphtheria and glanders in a solution of 1:250. Typhoid bacillus in 1:200. The growth of the anthrax bacillus and also the bacillus of diphtheria was prevented in culture solutions by a solution of 1:650.

Q. Has potash soap any disinfecting powers?

A. Yes; experiments have shown it to have considerable germicidal value. Jolles says that in experiments made by him with a soap, 67.44 per cent, of fat acids, 10.4 per cent of combined alkali and .041 per cent, of free alkali the following results were obtained: — The bacillus of typhoid fever was destroyed at 18 degrees C, by a one-per-cent solution in twenty-four hours, and by a six-per-cent solution in thirty minutes. These experiments show that scrubbing with soap and water is a reliable method of disinfecting surfaces. Solutions of potash, common lye, or of soda are also useful for certain purposes in domestic disinfection and scientific researches justify the continued use of the cleansing method which has heretofore been in use by careful housewives.

Q. How would you disinfect a room with formaldehyde and how much of the commercial article would you use for each one thousand cubic feet of space?

A. After closing every aperture of the room tightly by placing strips of paper over the cracks and crevices of the windows and doors, filling the keyhole with cotton, etc., I would hang sheets in the room and spray them with formaldehyde, using from ten to fifteen ounces to every thousand cubic feet of space, or I would use any of the generators now on the market for generating formaldehyde gas. A later method is the use of formaldehyde and permanganate of potash, six ounces of the latter to one pint of the former.

Q. What are considered the best generators?

A. There are a score or more on the market. Most of them are good. The question cannot be properly answered here.

Q. What are kresols?

A. A product of crude carbolic acid put up as proprietary preparations, known as tri-kresol, lysol, and by many other names.

Q. Of what are the various disinfectants composed?

A. Formaldehyde, bichloride of mercury, carbolic acid, kresol, chloride of lime, permanganate of potash and many other chemicals.

Q. What do you use to disinfect dwellings, apartments and clothing?

A. For dwellings or apartments, formaldehyde, sixteen ounces to one thousand cubic feet of space. Immerse clothing in a solution of chloride of lime, six ounces to a gallon of water, or expose them to the effect of chlorine, sulphurous acid or formaldehyde gas, for at least twenty-four hours.

Q. Do you always disinfect all contagious cases that come into your charge and do you instruct the family that it should be done and what they should use to do it with themselves?

A. I always disinfect all bodies dead of contagious diseases that come into my charge. I always instruct the family that it should be done, but never advise them to do it themselves, or instruct them as to what to use or how to proceed. It is the business of the undertaker or the Board of Health to disinfect premises.

Q. On what material and in what cases would you use the physical process of disinfection, what would you use, and what can you accomplish?

A. By physical process is meant without the use of chemicals. To disinfect sheets, pillow slips, bed spreads, napkins, towels or other cotton or linen goods that had been worn or slept in by a person afflicted with a contagious or infectious disease I would resort to boiling for at least thirty minutes. By this method I would accomplish the destruction of all germ life and render them innocuous. In smallpox or other highly contagious diseases I would burn all woolen goods, upholstered furniture or other material that could not be made safe by chemical disinfection.

Q. Can you safely guard yourself against contagious or infectious diseases, and if so, how?

A. No; one is never safe from infection while handling a contagious or infectious disease, but the danger can be mitigated by using due caution. In very dangerous cases a wet sponge over the mouth and nostrils would be advisable. In infectious cases such as septicemia, puerperal fever, erysipelas, and syphilis, the wearing of rubber gloves is advisable.

Q. What antiseptics do you carry in your case? In what strength and for what do you use them?

A. Formaldehyde 40 per cent, corrosive sublimate I:iooo, to disinfect myself, clothing, the body and if need be the premises. In using formaldehyde I reduce its strength when necessary.

Q. Should a body dead of an infectious or contagious disease be placed in a receiving vault after having been properly prepared for shipment? If not, why not?

A. It would do no harm, but might not be permitted through fear that the work had not been properly done, and beside this if the body is to be shipped it must be done within seventy-two hours after the time of death.

Q. Name some of the means of destroying germs.

A. Germs can be destroyed by sponging, spraying, or injecting with a fluid disinfectant, by the use of formaldehyde, chlorine or sulphurous acid gas, or by extreme heat in any form.

Q. Would a body wrapped in a sheet which had been saturated with a solution of bichloride of mercury, 1:1000, be considered disinfected?

A. No. The outside of the body, or at least as much of it as came in contact with the saturated sheet would be disinfected, but when unwrapped and allowed to dry the body would still be dangerous to the living.

Q. How do you mix carbolic acid to make a disinfectant?

A. Nineteen parts water to one of carbolic acid.

Q. What is the difference between formalin and formaldehyde?

A. Formaldehyde is the name of the original product. Formalin is a proprietary name. Formaldehyde gas is the gas contained in water, forty parts gas to sixty of water, known as commercial formaldehyde.

Q. In case you were without fluid or other disinfectant what could you substitute in its place if called upon to care for a dead body?

A. With the multitude of salesmen at present engaged in selling embalming fluid, one can hardly imagine such a case, but should it occur, you could use a saturated solution of salt and water, to which alcohol in any quantity could be added; both salt and alcohol being antiseptic, it would help to hold the body until you could do better, and would not interfere with embalming later. If you were near a drug store where a bottle of formaldehyde could be obtained, use that in solution of five per cent and you would probably have a well preserved body, though not a desirable color.

Q. What is the value of sulphate of iron (copperas) as a disinfectant?

A. According to Sternburg this salt does not destroy the vitality of disease germs, or the infecting power of material containing them. It is, nevertheless, a very valuable antiseptic, and its low price makes it one of the most available agents for the arrest of putrefaction.

Q. What disinfecting power has chloride of zinc?

A. Chloride of zinc is a useful antiseptic and one of the best deodorizers, but it is not to be depended upon as a means of destroying germs.

Q. What is the value of chloride of lime as a disinfectant?

A. It is considered one of the best and in many cases most available of disinfecting agents, on account of being an excellent deodorizer as well as germicide. It has been known to destroy typhoid bacillus in solution of one-half per cent, and in solution of two per cent is considered safe and reliable. Experiments made in the John Hopkins University, and confirmed by others made in Germany, induced the committee on disinfectants to give it the first place among drugs or chemicals as a disinfectant for excreta. According to experiments made by Bolton the typhoid bacillus and cholera spirillum were destroyed by a solution of 1:1000. Experiments made by Nisson in Koch's laboratory in 1890 proved that anthrax spores were destroyed in thirty minutes with a five-per-cent solution and in seventy minutes by a one-percent solution. These experiments proved that the typhoid bacillus and the cholera spirillum were destroyed with certainty in five minutes by a solution of 1:833, the anthrax bacillus in one minute by a solution of 1:1000, and other forms of bacteria in one minute by a 1:500 solution.

Q. What value has carbolic acid as a disinfectant?

A. It is one of the approved disinfectants and a five-percent solution will destroy almost any form of germ life in a short time.

Q. Is this a safe and reliable disinfectant for the excretions of the bowels in a typhoid fever case?

A. Yes; but chloride of lime is much better on account of its deodorizing qualities,

Q. What further advantages has carbolic acid as a disinfectant?

A. The committee on disinfectants says a five-per-cent solution of carbolic acid can be used instead of chloride of lime, the time of exposure to the action of the disinfectant being four hours. This recommendation is made in view of the fact that in those diseases in which it is most important to disinfect the excreta, the specific germ does not form spores. This is believed to be true of the typhoid bacillus, the spirillum of cholera, the bacillus of diphtheria, of glanders, and the streptococcus of erysipelas, and it has been shown by exact experiment that all of these pathogenic bacteria are destroyed in two hours by a one-per-cent solution of this agent.

Q. What is the best disinfecting solution for the sick room?

A. Chloride of lime on account of its deodorizing qualities, the rapidity of its action, and its cheapness.

Q. What is creolin?

A. A product of coal tar, believed to be a reliable disinfectant for most forms of germ life in solutions of from two to five per cent. The experiments of Eisenberg as given in Sternburg's bacteriology show that a solution of two per cent destroys all forms of bacteria in ten minutes. Esmarch found that it was especially fatal to the germs of cholera, destroying them in ten minutes at a strength of 1:1000, but other authorities state that in the presence of albumen its germicidal power is greatly diminished. As a deodorant it is considered superior to carbolic acid and on this account is preferred in the sick room.

Q. Name three antiseptic chemicals that are not considered safe and reliable disinfectants.

A. Chloride of zinc, permanganate of potash and sodium chloride.

Q. How would you produce sulphur dioxide for disinfecting apartments or rooms?

A. By saturating sulphur with alcohol and burning it in the presence of moisture.

Q. What will be the probable result of using only antiseptic chemicals in embalming a body?

A. It would probably keep for a short time; after that putrefaction would be likely to ensue.

Q. Name some disinfecting chemicals that are not deodorants.

A. Bichloride of mercury, formaldehyde and carbolic acid.

Q. Which will the vapor fumes of formaldehyde do while being used as a disinfectant, rise or fall?

A. They will rise.

Q. What disinfection of premises, if any, is necessary after death by consumption?

A. The premises should be properly disinfected with formaldehyde gas.

Q. What is the best disinfectant for infected clothing?

A. Formaldehyde gas. After using it, hang the clothing in an open yard and allow the sun to shine upon it and the air to pass through it.

Q. What, if any, danger from the dejecta of typhoid fever patients?

A. Danger of infection. It must either be burned or disinfected and then buried.

Q. What danger from the dejecta of cholera patients? Why?

A. Great danger, because the contents of the bowels contain the greatest number of germs. Burn, or disinfect and bury.

Q. What is considered the best disinfectant with which to inject the body? .

A. Formaldehyde,

Q. What is the object of disinfecting a body dead of a contagious or infectious disease?

A. To render it innocuous to the living.

Q. If infection is taking or receiving a poison, what effect will a disinfectant have?

A. It may destroy or retard the growth of poisonous germs.

Q. Name three disinfecting chemicals.

A. Bichloride of mercury, formaldehyde and chloride of lime.

Q. Are chemicals which will destroy a morbid odor considered strong enough to destroy the germs of contagion or infection as required by the State Boards of Health?

A. Some of them are. Chloride of lime is an excellent deodorizer and also a strong disinfectant, but most deodorizers are only mildly antiseptic.

Q. Name some good disinfectant and state proportion used to one gallon of water.

A. Bichloride of mercury, from one drachm to one-half ounce to a gallon of water, according to the use to be made of it.

Q. What is the value of formaldehyde as a disinfectant?

A. Formaldehyde gas is probably the best disinfectant for rooms or apartments known to science, and for that purpose is almost universally used.

Q. What disinfecting properties has sulphate of zinc?

A. None. It is slightly antiseptic and a strong dessicant.

Q. What do you know about hydrogen peroxide as a disinfectant?

A. It is a powerful antiseptic and germicide. It is used by physicians as an antiseptic in diphtheria, glandular swellings and suppurative inflammations. It will destroy the germs of typhoid fever at a strength of 1:1000.

Q. Of what antiseptic qualities is thymol possessed?

A. It is a powerful antiseptic and anaesthetic to the skin and mucous membrane. It is used principally by physicians as just as efficient and more agreeable than carbolic acid. It should be used as a spray at a strength of from a 1:2000 to 1:1000 solution.

Q. Why do you fumigate and disinfect apartments where death is caused by a contagious disease, and not where it results from a disease considered infectious only?

A. For the reason that the germs of an infectious disease are not spread by atmospheric diffusion. But there are many infectious diseases in which it is considered necessary to disinfect the sick room.

Q. Name some deodorant that may be used as a disinfectant.

A. Chloride of lime and permanganate of potash.

Q. The exterior of a body dead of a contagious disease should be washed with an approved disinfectant when being prepared for transportation. What disinfectant do you use? State proportions.

A. Bichloride of mercury; 1:1000.

Q. In sulphur fumigation, how much should be used for a room ten feet square?

A. From three to five pounds.

Q. To thoroughly disinfect a body dead of a contagious disease what parts should be filled with fluid by arterial injection?

A. All parts if possible.

Q. About how much fluid should be injected arterially to disinfect a body weighing 160 pounds?

A. That would depend largely on the kind of fluid used. If it was a strong disinfectant from three quarts to one gallon would be sufficient.

Q. What do we aim to sterilize or disinfect by cavity embalming?

A. The alimentary canal and other viscera.

Q. What is the best disinfectant for the discharges from patients? State proportion.

A. Chloride of lime; six ounces to a gallon of water.

Q. How is puerperal fever communicated?

A. By infection, either from the hands or infected instruments. The embalmer should be careful of abrasions on the hands while handling this or any other case of septic poisoning.

Q. What should be treated as infectious or contagious matter?

A. All discharges from the body of those afflicted with i contagious or infectious disease; faeces, urine, vomit and all discharges of the mouth and nostrils.

Q. What disinfectant do you use to disinfect your face, hands, hair, etc.?

A. Corrosive sublimate, 1:1000, or chloride of lime, one and one-half ounces to one quart of water.

Q. Soiled underwear, bed linen, pocket handkerchiefs, night robes, etc., should be boiled. What other precautions should be taken immediately after the articles are removed from the patient?

A. Put them to soak in an antiseptic solution; one-half drachm of corrosive sublimate to a gallon of water, or a five percent solution of formaldehyde.

Q. Name some disinfectants other than formaldehyde and state for what purpose you would use them and in what proportions.

A. Chloride of lime for faecal discharges, six ounces to a gallon of water, one quart for each discharge of the patient. Bichloride of mercury, one dram to a gallon of water for sponging bodies dead of contagious diseases.

Q. The discharges from a typhoid fever patient arc thrown upon ice on a pond while the temperature registers below zero. If the temperature does not rise for a week, will the water be infectious when the ice melts?

A. Yes; typhoid fever germs have been shown to be alive after having for several weeks been frozen in a cake of ice. Cold restrains the action of germ life, but seldom destroys the germs.

Q. What are the effects of an antiseptic on dead tissue?

A. To restrain the action of the pathogenic or putrefactive bacteria, to preserve the tissue for a short time, and to render it less dangerous to the living.

Q. Name two antiseptic chemicals.

A. Chloride of zinc and permanganate of potash.

Q. What are the effects of a disinfectant on dead tissue?

A. To destroy the germs of disease and putrefaction, to disinfect the tissue and preserve it for an indefinite period of time.

Q. Name two infectious diseases not considered contagious.

A. Typhoid fever and erysipelas.

Q. Are all embalming fluids considered safe and reliable disinfectants?

A. No; all embalming fluids are necessarily antiseptic, but they are not all reliable as disinfectants.

Q. How can an embalming fluid be made a disinfectant?

A. By adding bichloride of mercury, formaldehyde, or some other reliable disinfectant in proper proportions.

Q. How would you prepare a solution of bichloride of mercury to make a reliable disinfectant?

A. By adding one dram of corrosive sublimate to one gallon of water.

Q. How would you prepare a solution of carbolic acid to make an antiseptic?

A. By adding two parts of carbolic acid to ninety-eight parts of water.

Q. What is the principal cause of failure in attempted disinfection? How would you guard against it?

A. In disinfecting houses or apartments the principal cause of failure is not closing the rooms tightly; another cause is using too small a quantity of the disinfectant. I would see that all cracks and crevices were closed by pasting strips of paper over them and would use even more than the prescribed amount of disinfecting material.

Q. How would you disinfect a house or room with sulphur? How much does it require?

A. After preparing the house or apartment, I would place three or four pounds of sulphur for every thousand cubic feet of space to be disinfected in an old vessel and cover it with charcoal, then saturate the whole with alcohol, and place this vessel inside another of larger size partially filled with water and apply a lighted match. This will give sulphur dioxide, or sulphurous acid gas, and moisture sufficient to make it effective.

Q. What is the best means of disinfecting a home, and what diseases require it?

A. Formaldehyde gas. Smallpox, diphtheria, Asiatic cholera, scarlet fever, scarletina, anthrax, or any other disease known to be contagious.

Q. When bichloride of mercury is the only disinfectant contained in the embalming fluid used in a contagious case, are you sure the body is thoroughly disinfected?

A. If a sufficient quantity were used there would be little or no doubt of it; but bichloride of mercury brought in contact with albumen forms albuminate of mercury, which is not a disinfectant, and the usual quantity might not bring about the desired result.

Q. What is the least possible time a room should be left exposed under proper conditions as to heat, moisture, etc., where sixteen ounces of formaldehyde to each thousand cubic feet of space has been used, in diseases such as scarlet fever and diphtheria?

A. At least six hours. If convenient to do so, leave the room closed for from twelve to twenty-four hours.

Q. After a sufficient time has elapsed what would you do?

A. Open the doors and windows and admit air and sunshine. The value of these supplementary measures cannot be overestimated.

Q. What are the first duties of the embalmer when called to a home where death has been caused by a contagious disease?

A. Advise the family to have the room as well as the body disinfected at once; warn them not to kiss the remains, and to keep away from the room as much as possible. A weak or sickly member of the household should be particularly cautioned, as such are most susceptible to the disease.

Q. What are germicides?

A. The same as disinfectants; chemicals that will destroy germ life.

Q. What is the most effective disinfectant for the woodwork of an infected dwelling?

A. Bichloride of mercury.

Q. How strong would you make it for this purpose?

A. One part to five hundred, or two drachms to one gallon of water.

Q. Name the contagious and infectious diseases that are most prevalent in the Northern States.

A. Smallpox, scarlet fever, typhoid fever, diphtheria, measles, and pneumonia, also the disease known as la grippe.

Q. Name those most peculiar to the Southern States.

A. Yellow fever, typhus fever and malaria are the principle ones peculiar to that section, but there are many diseases that are not confined to ahy particular section of the country.

Q. Would you embalm a body in the same way for disinfection as for preservation?

A. The same, except that I would be sure to use a fluid that was a safe disinfectant, and a sufficient quantity in doing my arterial work to reach air of the tissues of the body, and would take the extra precaution of sponging the body, washing out the apertures and packing them with cotton.

Q. Do you observe any difference in the treatment of a body dead of a contagious and infectious disease? If so, what?

A. There are some infectious diseases in which it would not be necessary to sponge the outside of the body, or be very particular about washing out and packing the apertures, but most infectious diseases should be treated as contagious.

Q. To what extent may a sickroom be disinfected while occupied, and how may it be done?

A. It may be disinfected to a certain extent by hanging sheets in the room and spraying them with a solution of chloride of zinc, which, while not a safe disinfectant, is antiseptic and a good deodorizer; a solution of chloride of lime may be used for disinfecting all excretions from the patient, and bichloride of mercury in proportions of 1:1000 may be used for woodwork or furniture that is not upholstered.

Q. What is the difference between an antiseptic, a disinfectant and a deodorizer?

A. A disinfectant destroys germ life; an antiseptic restrains the growth and multiplication of germs; a deodorizer destroys pad odors. Bichloride of mercury is a disinfectant; permanganate of potash is an antiseptic and also a deodorizer; chloride of zinc is an excellent deodorizer.

Q. If septic is a poison, what effect will an antiseptic have?

A. It will retard the growth of the poisonous germs, and prevent their multiplication and consequent fatal poisoning.

Q. Name four contagious diseases, and describe the manner in which they may be severally communicated.

A. Smallpox, from a person at any stage of the disease; scarlet fever, probably communicable at any stage, but more dangerous when the body commences to peal; diphtheria, communicated by germs from the saliva (probably the whole body is affected); measles, by contact with the body or the atmosphere of the sick room.

Q. How would you disinfect the hands after having cared for a body dead of a contagious disease?

A. Remove all visible dirt from beneath and around the nails and brush thoroughly with soap and hot water, wash the hands in alcohol and then, for about a minute, in a two percent solution of carbolic acid or a 1:1000 solution of bichloride of mercury.

Q. Give another method of disinfecting the hands?

A. Sternburg gives the following formula: First, cleanse the finger nails of all visible dirt with a knife or nail cleaner; second, brush the hands for three minutes with hot water and potash soap; third, wash for half a minute in a three-per-cent solution of carbolic acid and subsequently in a 1:2000 solution of mercuric chloride; fourth, rub the spaces beneath the nails and around their margins with iodoform gauze wet with a five-per-cent solution of carbolic acid. Welch gives the following directions: The nails should be kept short and clean, the hands washed thoroughly for a few minutes in soap and water, the water being as warm as can be comfortably borne and frequently changed; a brush sterilized by steam should be used and the excess of soap washed off with water; the hands should now be immersed from one to two minutes in a warm saturated solution of permanganate of potash and rubbed thoroughly with a sterilized swab. They should then be placed in a warm solution of oxalic acid, where they should remain until discoloration of the permanganate occurs. They should then be washed with sterilized salt solution or water, then immersed for two minutes in sublimate solution, 1:500.

Q. What are the most useful agents for the destruction of spore containing infectious material?

A. Complete destruction by burning; steam under pressure; 221 degrees F., for ten minutes; boiling in water for half an hour; chloride of lime, a four-per-cent solution; corrosive sublimate, 1:500.

Q. What are the most useful disinfectants for the disinfection of material containing microorganisms where spores are not believed to be present?

A. Complete destruction by burning; if valuable, and it can be done without destroying the value, boiling in water for one-half hour or exposure to dry heat, 212 degrees to 230 degrees F., immersion in a two-per-cent solution of chloride of lime, immersion in a 1:2000 solution of bichloride of mercury, a three-per-cent solution of carbolic acid, or a ten-percent solution of chloride of zinc, and afterward boiling for half an hour.

Q. What are the best disinfectants for privy vaults?

A. Bichloride of mercury, 1:500; carbolic acid, five per cent; chloride of lime, six ounces to a gallon of water; for the disinfecting and deodorizing of the surface of organic material, chloride of lime in powder.

Q. What disinfectants were recommended by the committee of the American Public Health Association for clothing, bedding, etc.?

A. Destruction by fire if of little value. Boiling for at least half an hour; immersion in a solution of mercuric chloride of the strength of 1:2000 for four hours; and immersion in a two-percent solution of carbolic acid for two hours.

Q. What recommendations were made for disinfecting outer garments of wool, silk and similar articles, which would be injured by immersion in boiling water or in a disinfecting solution?

A. First, exposure in a suitable apparatus to a current of steam for ten minutes; second, exposure to dry heat At a temperature of 230 degrees F. for two hours.

Q. How would you disinfect mattresses and blankets soiled by the discharges of the sick?

A. The committee's recommendations are first, the destruction by fire; second, exposure to superheated steam of 221 degrees F., for ten minutes, mattresses to have the covers removed or freely opened; third, immersion in boiling water for half an hour.

Q. What recommendations were made in relation to the disinfection of furniture, articles of wood, porcelain and leather?

A. Washing, several times repeated, in a two-per-cent solution of carbolic acid.

Q. What recommendations were made for disinfecting the persons of those in attendance on patients sick of a contagious disease, or of convalescents?

A. The hands and general surface of the body should be washed with a solution of chlorinated soda diluted with nine parts of water, carbolic acid, two-per-cent solution, or mercuric chloride, 1:1000.

Q. What disinfectants were recommended for the dead?

A. Envelope the body in a sheet thoroughly saturated with a four-per-cent solution of chloride of lime, mercuric chloride in solution 1:500, and carbolic acid in solution, five per cent.

Q. Would this be necessary if the body were embalmed and properly disinfected?

A. No.

Q. How would you disinfect hospitals and sick rooms while occupied?

A. The committee recommend that all surfaces be washed with mercuric chloride in solution, 1:1000, or carbolic acid in solution, two per cent,

Q. What recommendations are made in relation to their disinfection when vacated?

A. To fumigate with sulphur dioxide for twelve hours, burning at least three pounds of sulphur for every thousand cubic feet of air space in the room, then wash all surfaces with one of the above-mentioned disinfecting solutions, and afterward with hot water and soap, and finally throw open doors and windows and ventilate freely.

Q. Is this method of disinfecting practised at the present time?

A. No, since the advent of formaldehyde, sulphur dioxide is seldom or never used, washing the surfaces with bichloride of mercury, however, and thorough ventilation are still to be recommended.

Q. Is it necessary to destroy the contents of the home after a scourge of smallpox to insure future safety of its inmates not immune to the disease?

A. Not strictly necessary, but advisable as to at least a part of the furniture.

Q. If it were your home and your circumstances would not permit of the loss, what part of the contents would you try to preserve and what method would you employ?

A. All crockery, glass and silverware, all wooden furniture, all bedding, towels, table linen, napkins, and underwear composed of cotton or linen. I would wash all wooden wear with a 1:500 solution of bichloride of mercury, all crockery or silverware with a fifteen-per-cent solution of formaldehyde, and immerse all cotton or linen articles in boiling water for at least thirty minutes.

Q. How do you disinfect sponges, towels, instruments and cooling boards used in diphtheria?

A. By boiling cloths and towels for a period not less than thirty minutes; soaking sponges in formaldehyde; sponging the cooling board with a 1:500 solution of bichloride of mercury; sterilizing instruments with steam, or immerse them for thirty minutes in a fifteen-per-cent solution of formaldehyde.

Q. In what cases is vomit believed to be infectious?

A. In all cases of cholera, diphtheria, yellow and scarlet fevers, the National Committee recommend that all vomited material be disinfected.

Q. In what cases is it necessary to disinfect the sputum?

A. In tuberculosis, diphtheria, scarlet fever and pneumonia.

Q. How should this be done?

A. With an approved disinfectant or by burning before it is dried. The latter is to be recommended.

Q. Should the urine voided by patients sick of an infectious disease be disinfected?

A. Yes, mix with a solution of chloride of lime, six ounces to one gallon of water, using one pint to each discharge before emptying it into the sewer.

Q. What special treatment should be given a body dead of diphtheria?

A. Thoroughly sponge the body with an approved disinfectant; cleanse and sterilize all orifices, and pack them with cotton; embalm the body arterially and fill the serous cavities, using an embalming fluid known to be a disinfectant. Disinfect by burning or boiling all articles, such as towels, napkins, cloths or bedding that has been in contact with the body or in the room.

Q. How would you disinfect a body dead of consumption?

A. The same as in diphtheria; in addition to the treatment given there, the air cells of the lungs should always be injected.

Q. Should pneumonia be treated as a contagious disease? How treat it?

A. Yes; it is classed as contagious. Treat it in the same manner as tuberculosis.

Q. How would you treat a body dead of yellow fever? Can such a case be shipped?

A. It is probable that the germs of this disease could be destroyed by the use of any standard disinfectant, but the health officers would probably not allow a body dead of yellow fever to be held long enough to be embalmed. It is much more probable that they would order the body wrapped in a sheet saturated with bichloride of mercury and buried at once. In some states the Board of Health permits the shipping of bodies dead of yellow fever when prepared by a licensed embalmer. When this is done, first sponge the body with a solution of corrosive sublimate, 1:500, or two drams to a gallon of water, then sterilize all orifices with a like solution and pack with cotton saturated with it. Embalm arterially, adding a sufficient quantity of formaldehyde, or other chemicals, to make the fluid a safe disinfectant, and fill all serous cavities. Then bandage in a layer of absorbent cotton one inch thick, and wrap in a sheet, securely fastened and covering the body completely. Enclose in an air-tight, zinc, tin, copper or lead-lined coffin or iron casket, all joints and seams hermetically sealed and enclosed in a strong, tight wooden box.

Q. What special treatment should be given a case of typhoid fever?

A. In addition to arterial embalming, wash out the apertures with a disinfectant and pack them tightly with cotton, sterilize the alimentary canal and sponge the surface of the body. As the germs are supposed to be largely confined to the alimentary canal and abdominal viscera, the thorough sterilizing of these parts of the body is very important.

Q. If required to remove a body from one cemetery to another that had died of a dangerously contagious disease how would you proceed?

A. I would first obtain a permit to do so from the proper authorities. Then see that myself and my assistants were properly dressed for the occasion. I would then provide myself with about two gallons of a 1:500 solution of corrosive sublimate, and when near to the box sprinkle the soil with this solution and, after they have been removed, spray the box and casket or coffin. When the receptacle has been opened, disinfect the remains in the same way and remove in a metallic lined casket, coffin or box.

Chemistry

Q. What is chemistry?

A. It is that science which treats of atoms and molecules and teaches those rules which govern their changes and combinations.

Q. What is organic chemistry?

A. Organic chemistry treats of carbon and its compounds, of cells and their structure; also of the substances involved in the transformation processes of life and decay.

Q. What is an atom?

A. An atom is an ultimate unit of matter; that which cannot be further divided.

Q. What is a molecule?

A. The smallest quantity of any material substance which can exist uncombined.

Q. What are the chemical constituents of the human body?

A. Oxygen, carbon, hydrogen and nitrogen are present in all the organic tissues of the body, and constitute about 97 per cent of the whole structure. Sulphur, phosphorus, chlorine, fluorine, silica, potassium, sodium, magnesium, calcium and iron are necessary constituents, but in very small quantities.

Q. What part of the human body is water?

A. About eight-tenths.

Q. What is oxygen?

A. Oxygen is a colorless, tasteless gas, which constitutes about one-fifth of the atmosphere, about one-half of the bulk and about eight-ninths of the weight of water, three-fourths of organized bodies and about one-half the crust of the earth.

Q. What is hydrogen?

A. A gaseous element occurring in nature combined with oxygen in the form of water. Hydrogen has no taste or color and the pure gas no odor.

Q. What is carbon?

A. A non-metal, occurring in nature in various forms, such as diamond, graphite or black lead and charcoal, also an element of coal and similar substances. The acid gaseous product has the composition of $CO2$, carbon dioxide, commonly known as carbonic acid gas. It is a colorless gas, having a specific gravity of 1.52. It is soluble in cold water and possesses a pungent smell and an acid taste. Inhaled it destroys animal life by asphyxiation. Graphite is a soft black, shiny solid, which is soft and soapy to the touch. Pure graphite is carbon.

Q. What is nitrogen?

A. Nitrogen is one of the non-metallic elements, gaseous at ordinary temperature, a component element of ammonia, various acids and a great number of animal and vegetable tissues. It forms 80 per cent of the air and is most active in combination with oxygen.

Q. What is sulphur?

A. It is a non-metallic element distinguished by a yellow color and crystaline properties. It is one of the acid elements, and unites with oxygen to form the most powerful acid radicals.

Q. What is phosphorus?

A. A non-metal existing in three allotropic forms. Yellow phosphorus is of waxy consistency, soluble in carbon disulphide. Red phosphorus is pulverent and insoluble. Metallic phosphorus has a metallic lustre, and is insoluble and inert at ordinary temperatures; it is an essential element in brain, nerve and bone tissue.

Q. What is chlorine?

A. A non-metallic element, at ordinary temperature a greenish yellow gas, prepared by decomposing sodium chloride. A valuable antiseptic.

Q. What is fluorine?

A. One of the elements. It has not been isolated, but is probably a gas. All the salts are highly corrosive and in their full strength poisonous.

Q. What is silica?

A. The oxide of silicon. It occurs in nature and in the mineral form, of which sea sand is a familiar example.

Q. What is potassium?

A. A metallic element of silvery lustre, alkaline and characterized by an intense affinity for oxygen.

Q. What is sodium?

A. A metal of the alkaline group, characterized by a strong affinity for oxygen. It has a silver white lustre, and is softer than lead. It decomposes water, forming sodium hydrate.

Q. What is magnesium?

A. One of the alkaline metals represented in medicine by several mineral and organic salts. The sulphate occurs in sea water and many rocks and soils.

Q. What is calcium?

A. A brilliant silver white metal, the basis of lime and limestone, characterized by strong affinity for oxygen and isolated with great difficulty; best known in the form of calcium oxide, quicklime.

Q. What are cells?

A. Cells are nucleated masses of protoplasm, usually with cell walls, which enter into a structure, and on which depend form, shape, and consistence.

Q. What is life?

A. Life is that form of energy on which the phenomena exhibited by organized beings depends, from the protoplasm of first vitalized essence to the highly elaborated and extremely complicated animal body.

Q. What is death?

A. Death is the withdrawal and absence of that energy.

Q. What is an organ?

A. An organ is a complexus of similar or dissimilar cells, which unite to perform a certain function.

Q. When life ceases what changes take place?

A. When life ceases chemical action begins, which if not arrested will continue until the lately organized body returns to its inorganic elements.

Q. When do these chemical changes commence?

A. In some cases chemical changes are begun while the body is still alive, in others all visible change may be delayed for some time.

Q. What are these chemical changes usually called?

A. Fermentation and putrefaction.

Q. What do you understand by fermentation?

A. The combustion of the proteids. The union of carbon with oxygen, forming carbon dioxide, or what is more commonly known as carbonic acid gas, the setting free of hydrogen gas and the union of the latter with sulphur.

Q. What is the result of this chemical condition in a dead body?

A. The phenomenon popularly, but improperly, called purging.

Q. What is putrefaction?

A. Putrefaction may be defined as a condition resulting in the fermentation of albuminous tissues caused by the invasion and multiplication of microorganisms known as putrefactive bacteria.

Q. How can the process of putrefaction be arrested?

A. By the removal of all putrefactive material possible in the dead body and the introduction or injection of preservative and disinfecting chemicals to destroy the germs of putrefaction and preserve and harden the tissues.

Q. Name some of the chemicals which when properly combined will resist the process of putrefaction.

A. Arsenic, bichloride of mercury, formaldehyde, carbolic acid, chloride of zinc, sulphate of zinc, sodium chloride, alcohol and boracic acid.

Q. What chemicals enter into the composition of an embalming fluid?

A. All those above named, in different combination, and many others.

Q. Name a disinfecting chemical, a solution of which should never be made in a copper, lead or tin dipper, and state reasons.

A. Bichloride of mercury because of its corrosive qualities.

Q. Name some of the chemicals that have a tendency to prevent coagulation of the blood.

A. Sodium chlorides, magnesium sulphates and sodium sulphates.

Q. What chemicals enter into the composition of a bleacher?

A. Alcohol, sulphate of zinc, chloride of zinc, camphor and other chemicals.

Q. How would you prepare one gallon of a 1:1000 solution of bichloride of mercury? A 1:500 solution?

A. For a 1:1000 solution add one dram of corrosive sublimate to one gallon of water. For a 1:500 solution two drams to a gallon of water.

Q. What strength should be used for washing fabrics and what for washing woodwork?

A. A 1:1000 solution for washing fabrics, and a 1:500 for woodwork.

Q. How would you prepare a smaller quantity of each?

A. To make one quart of a 1:1000 solution add one-fourth dram or fifteen grains to a quart of water, and for a 1:500 solution twice the quantity or one-half dram. For a pint of a 1:1000 solution add one-eighth dram to a pint of water, and for 1:500 solution one-fourth dram.

Q. How much water would you add to a pint of formaldehyde to make a 40 per cent solution?

A. What is known as commercial formaldehyde contains forty parts formaldehyde gas and sixty parts of water, and no water is needed, as it is already a 40 per cent solution.

Q. How would you prepare a 10 per cent solution? An 8 per cent solution? A 5 per cent solution? A 2 per cent solution? A 1 per cent solution?

A. To prepare a 10 per cent solution add three pints of water to one of formaldehyde. To make an 8 per cent solution add four parts of water to one of formaldehyde. To make a 5 per cent solution add seven parts of water to one of formaldehyde. To make a 2 per cent solution add nineteen parts of water to one of formaldehyde. To make a 1 per cent solution add thirty-nine parts of water to one of formaldehyde.

Q. How would you produce sulphurous acid gas.

A. Take a quantity of sulphur and place it in a vessel, cover it with charcoal and saturate the whole with alcohol and apply a lighted match.

Q. How would you produce chlorine gas for disinfecting a room or apartments?

A. Place a quantity of chloride of lime in an old vessel and dampen it with water, spread over this about four ounces of muriatic acid far each pound of chloride of lime and the result will be chlorine gas.

Section III - The Essentials of Embalming

Q. What is embalming? Give a brief history of the art.

A. Embalming is the preservation and disinfection of dead bodies by the intelligent use of chemicals, which is today the injection of the arteries and when necessary the cavities of dead bodies with preparations of disinfecting and preserving chemicals, for the purpose of rendering them inoccuous and inoffensive to the living, also pleasant to look upon. Of ancient embalming very little is known, and to attempt to give a history of it, ever so brief, would be out of place in a work of this kind. The first man to practise embalming to any extent in this country was Dr. Holmes, late of Brooklyn, N. Y., who practised it in a crude way in the army during the Civil War, embalming the bodies of many of the officers and men for transportation to their homes in the north. In 1880 Prof. J. H. Clark, now of Cincinnati, commenced the business of teaching embalming, a profession in which he has been engaged since that time. He was followed by many other teachers of the art, and is to be honored as the founder of embalming schools.

Q. How soon after death should a body be embalmed?

A. Many would say as soon as may be after the fact that death has taken place has been established, but my own opinion is that the work is more satisfactory if the body is placed on an incline and the blood allowed to gravitate to the dependent parts for several hours before embalming.

Q. What is the meaning of the word embalm?

A. To preserve with balm or balsam; to impregnate with aromatics in order to prevent putrefaction. The modern meaning is, of course, to preserve with chemicals.

Q. Name the various methods of embalming and state how they differ.

A. Strictly speaking, there is but one method of embalming a dead body, which is to raise and inject an artery. However, as this method is not always successful and as many so-called embalmers are unable to raise an artery, other methods of preserving bodies are resorted to, and are called needle and cavity embalming. By arterial embalming all the tissues of the body are reached by the fluid, provided there are no obstructions in the arteries. Should there be obstructions in an artery supplying an organ, and there often is, that tissue may be left without a supply of preservatives; therefore, intelligent embalmers resort to needle and cavity work as a means of guarding against failure. Cavity embalming is the injection of the serous cavities of the body for the purpose of surrounding the viscera therein contained with fluid, hoping to thus temporarily preserve them, which it may or may not do. Cavity work, then, should be known as an expedient and not as a process. Needle embalming, so-called, is the injection of the sinuses of the dura mater and through these the vessels of the brain, thereby preserving that organ. The fluid thus, injected may find its way into a part of the viscera by venous circulation, and possibly, but not probably, into the tissues of the whole body, by taking the course of the pulmonary circulation.

Arterial Embalming

Q. What is arterial embalming?

A. The injection of preservative and disinfecting chemicals into the vascular system for the purpose of disinfecting and preserving the tissues of the body.

Q. What means have you of knowing if the vascular system has been injected?

A. No one can tell when a perfect circulation of the embalming fluid has been obtained. The raising of the superficial vessels of the face, hands or feet will indicate a circulation in those parts, but the operator must bear in mind that this is no proof that the fluid has penetrated to all parts of the body. An obstruction of the coeliac axis, for instance, would prevent the fluid from finding its way into any of those organs supplied by its three divisions, the liver, stomach or spleen. Hardening of the flesh or bleaching of the skin would indicate that the fluid had penetrated to the parts affected.

Q. What is accomplished by embalming?

A. If the work is properly done the body is preserved, disinfected and made pleasant to the sight.

Q. Is embalming a benefit to the living?

A. Certainly; it makes the body inoccuous, odorless and pleasant to look upon.

Q. How would you supply the vascular system with fluid?

A. By raising and injecting an artery.

Q. What quantity of fluid is necessary for effective embalming in the average case?

A. About three quarts.

Q. In case you do both arterial and cavity work, which do you do first?

A. Arterial, as there is always a possibility of rupturing blood vessels in doing cavity work.

Q. Name three ways of embalming a dead body and give a description of each.

A. Arterial, cavity and so-called needle embalming. A description of each process is given in another part of this work.

Q. In the process of arterial embalming, what instruments are used? State the use you make of each instrument.

A. Scalpel, aneurism hook, arterial tube, separator, forceps, scissors, aspirator and injector, and sometimes a needle. The scalpel is used for cutting, the separator for opening the sheath and afterwards to rest the artery on, forceps for raising vessels or fascia, the aneurism hook for raising the vessel, the arterial tube through which to inject the fluid, scissors for cutting thread, aspirator for drawing blood, should it be necessary to do so, and a needle for closing the incision.

Q. Locate the following arteries: Common carotid, brachial, radial, ulnar and femoral.

A. The common carotid is in the neck, between the sterno mastoid muscle and the trachea; the brachial in the upper arm, extending along the base of the biceps muscle; the radial in the forearm, extending from the .bifurcation of the brachial to the deep palmar arch; the ulnar is in the forearm, extending from the bifurcation of the brachial to the superficial palmar arch; the femoral in the thigh, commencing at Poupart's ligament and extending to the popliteal space.

Q. Explain fully the best method of raising and injecting the common carotid artery.

A. Make an incision just above the junction of the clavicle and sternum, between the sterno-mastoid muscle and the trachea, cut through the skin, fat and cervical fascia, insert the index finger in the wound and move it backward and forward between the trachea and the muscle (the artery being large and its walls thick, it can easily be located by the touch). Then, using the separator, release the artery from the sheath and raise it to the surface with the aneurism hook.

Q. What are the functions of the superior and inferior mesenteric arteries?

A. The superior mesenteric artery supplies the whole of the small intestines except a small part of the duodenum, also the caecum, ascending and transverse colon. The inferior mesenteric artery supplies the descending colon, and the sigmoid flexure.

Q. How can arterial embalming be done when the body has been posted and arteries severed?

A. Ligature the severed vessels whenever it can be done effectually. When this cannot be accomplished, embalm in sections, pack the viscera in hardening compound and do hypodermic work. See post mortem and mutilated cases.

Q. What are positive indications of a thorough circulation of fluid in a body embalmed arterially?

A. There are no positive indications of a thorough circulation. The return of fluid through the veins, the distension of the superficial vessels, and the hardening of the tissues, are positive indications of a circulation in a particular part only.

Q. If on cutting for the brachial artery you failed to find it, what would you do?

A. I can hardly imagine such a case, but should I be troubled to locate the brachial artery I would raise the axillary, which lies in the axillary space at the base of the arm pit muscle.

Q. How would you positively distinguish an artery from a vein?

A. The walls of the arteries are very thick as compared with veins, owing to the large quantity of muscular tissue in their composition; therefore, if an artery be rolled between the fingers it will easily be seen to be a thick muscular tube; but owing to the fact that the walls of veins sometimes become thickened this is not a positive test. The only places in the body where the embalmer is liable to mistake a vein for an artery are in the brachial space and Scarpa's triangle. The brachial artery is accompanied by two small veins, one on either side of the vessel, called Venae comites or brachial veins, together with the median nerve, all of which are enclosed in a sheath at the base of the biceps muscle. The basilic vein, the only one that can possibly be mistaken for the brachial artery usually extends along the inner border of the triceps muscle, and has no accompanying veins. Should the embalmer be in doubt as to the vessel he has secured, he has only to ascertain if it is accompanied by a small vein on either side, and if he finds them he can rest assured that he has the brachial artery. In Scarpa's triangle the femoral artery and vein are in the same sheath, the vein lying posterior to the artery and separated from that vessel by a membranous partition. Its walls are always thin and it usually contains blood, and cannot be mistaken for the artery. But the long saphenous vein frequently passes directly over the course of the femoral artery and its walls are sometimes thickened so that it might be mistaken for the artery. If the embalmer is in doubt he can easily make certain by ascertaining if there are two vessels in the same sheath; if not, it is not the artery, and he should continue to search until he finds the conditions named.

Q. Give the landmarks by which you locate the femoral artery.

A. The artery lies in the center of Scarpa's triangle, which is bounded on the outside by the sartorius muscle, on the inside by the adductor longus, and above by Poupart's ligament. With these anatomical guides in mind there should be no trouble in locating the vessel.

Q. Why do you inject an artery instead of a vein?

A. Most veins have valves while arteries have none. Arteries are usually empty. Veins always contain blood.

Q. Name the artery of the neck used in embalming.

A. The common carotid.

Q. Name the artery of the thigh used in embalming.

A. The femoral.

Q. Name the arteries of the arm used in embalming.

A. The brachial in the upper arm, often the radial and sometimes the ulnar in the forearm.

Q. Why do you inject an artery toward the heart and not from it?

A. All systemic arteries originate in the great trunk artery of the body, the great aorta, which arises at the left ventricle of the heart; when injecting toward that organ, I am forcing the fluid to the aorta, which through its branches and sub-branches conveys it to all of the tissues.

Q. Give the linear guide for locating the radial artery.

A. A line drawn from the center of the condyles of the humerus (elbow joint) to the inner side of the wrist joint will be directly over the course of the radial artery.

Q. Give the anatomical guides for locating the radial artery.

A. The anatomical guides are the supinator longus and the flexor carpi radialis muscles (the two muscles on the thumb side of the forearm); the artery lies between them.

Q. How would you proceed to raise the radial artery?

A. The radial artery, the smaller division of the brachial, lies between the two muscles on the thumb side of the forearm. The tendon of the inside muscle is plainly visible and furnishes an excellent guide for locating the vessel, as it lies between this and the outside tendon, which shows less plainly from the fact that it lies flat on the radius or wrist bone. When about to raise this artery the embalmer should grasp the hand, not the arm, and holding it at a right angle to the body extend the arm fully and the depression between the tendons of the muscles becomes apparent. After selecting the point for raising the vessel hold the arm with the left hand, and the scalpel in the right, and make an incision about three-fourths of an inch in length, cutting through the skin, superficial fascia and fat. Now clear away the fascia and fatty tissue with the separator or the handle of the aneurism hook. Then open the wound with the fingers and the artery will be plainly visible, and you have only to raise it to the surface.

Q. At what point should the artery be raised?

A. About three inches above the wrist joint.

Q. Are there any veins in the same sheath with this artery?

A. Yes, its accompanying veins, called venae comites, but they are very small and are usually attached to the artery, and should be allowed to remain so; they will give the embalmer no trouble.

Q. Are there any veins in that part of the arm where the radial artery is situated that might mislead the embalmer?

A. Yes; the radial vein, a superficial vessel. It is quite large, is formed by radicals on the radial side of the hand, and ascends along the thumb side of the forearm to the bend of the elbow. This vessel has been known to cross the course of the radial artery and has sometimes been mistaken for that vessel, but this phenomenon is unusual and the mistake can easily be detected as it is more superficial than the artery and has no accompanying vessels.

Q. Give the linear guides for locating the brachial artery?

A. Holding the arm, palm upward, at a right angle to the body, draw a string from a point a little to the outside of the axillary space to the center of the elbow joint. This will give the position of the vessel in its upper and middle thirds. In the lower third the artery will be found about half an inch to the outer side of the string.

Q. Give the anatomical guides for locating the brachial artery?

A. The anatomical guides are the biceps muscle above and triceps below the vessel, together with the median nerve, which is in the same sheath with the artery.

Q. How would you proceed to raise the brachial artery?

A. The brachial artery is a continuation of the axillary and extends along the base of the biceps muscle to a point one-half inch below the bend of the elbow. It is enclosed in the sheath with the median nerve and its two accompanying veins. The basilic vein is also in the same sheath, but is separated from the brachial artery by the bicipital fascia. The vessel may be raised in any part of its course, as it is superficial throughout its length. When about to raise this vessel the operator should seat himself in a chair beside the subject, and, holding the arm, palm upward, at right angles to the body, proceed to locate the point at which to make the incision. Most embalmers choose the middle third of the muscle. If possible, he should locate the median nerve, with the ends of his fingers. Having cut through the skin, superficial fascia and fat, he will be in contact with the deep fascia, which forms the sheath enclosing the artery, nerve and accompanying veins. Open the sheath with a scalpel or by tearing it with the aneurism hook. Clear the fascia from the artery and other contents of the sheath; the vessel wanted will usually be found just beneath the nerve; push the nerve to one side and raise the artery to the surface.

Q. Is there any danger of mistaking the basilic vein for the brachial artery?

A. Not if the vessel first named is in its normal condition, as its walls are very thin, making it easy to distinguish between the veins and the arteries, the walls of which are comparatively very thick. But it frequently happens that the walls of the basilic vein become thickened, making that vessel resemble an artery so closely as to deceive an expert, unless he is very careful. The danger of mistaking this vessel for the brachial artery can be easily overcome in two ways. First, draw the arm tight and place the fingers at the basfe of the biceps muscles and feel for the median nerve. If found there, the vessel accompanying it is the brachial artery. If still in doubt look closely and see if there are two small veins, one on either side, accompanying the vessel; if so, all doubts should be removed.

Q. Give the linear guide for locating the common carotid artery.

A. A string drawn from the mastoid process in the temporal bone (the prominence of bone behind the ear) to the junction of the sternum and clavicle (collar and breast bone) will give the course of the common carotid artery.

Q. Give the anatomical guide for locating the common carotid artery.

A. The anatomical guides are the sterno mastoid muscle and the trachea.

Q. How would you proceed to raise the common carotid artery?

A. Make a transverse incision about three-fourths of an inch in length at a point midway between the sterno mastoid muscle and the trachea and near the top of the breast bone; cut through the skin, fat and cervical fascia, and if necessary sever the muscle from its attachment to the breast bone. Then introduce the finger between the sterno mastoid muscle and the trachea and locate the vessel by the sense of touch. The walls of the artery are very thick, making it easy to feel the vessel lying in its sheath between the organs previously mentioned. Having located the artery, hold it under the index finger of the left hand and with the right sever the sheath either with the separator or with the handle of the aneurism hook; when cleared from the surrounding tissue, raise it to the surface.

Q. Give the linear guide for locating the femoral artery.

A. Draw a string from the anterior superior spinous process of the ilium (sharp point of the hip bone) to the pubic bone (frontal bone of the pelvis). Then double the string, which will give you the center of Poupart's ligaments. From this point draw the string to the inside of the knee joint and it is exactly over the course of the femoral artery.

Q. Give the anatomical guide for locating the femoral artery.

A. The anatomical guides for locating this vessel are the sartorius muscle on the outside, the adductor longus on the inside and Poupart's ligament above, which organs, by their position, form what is known as Scarpa's triangle in the upper portion of the thigh. In the midst of this triangular space lies the femoral artery. An excellent way to use this guide for locating the vessel is to place the tips of the fingers in the depression formed by the two muscles, as in this way the course of the artery can easily be traced.

Q. How would you proceed to raise the femoral artery?

A. Make an incision in the center of Scarpa's triangle, at a point about one-half inch below Poupart's ligament, cut through the skin, fat and fascia lata, and the artery will be found enclosed in its sheath together with the femoral vein, the latter vessel being separated from the former by a membranous partition. In all bodies having little surplus flesh the artery at this point will be found to be very superficially located. While opening the sheath care should be taken not to rupture the vein, as it always contains blood, an effusion of which will be very embarrassing to the embalmer. Having separated the artery from the vein, raise it to the surface.

Q. What causes a body to purge by injecting it arterially?

A. It is impossible to answer this question definitely. The purging may be caused by pressure of gas, which should have been relieved. If it is the embalming fluid that is escaping, it is probably caused by a rupture of the bronchial or pulmonary circulation. If it is the products of fermentation escaping from the stomach or lungs, the cause is pressure of gas.

Q. Can a body be arterially embalmed if death is caused by childbirth and milk-leg, before the child is born?

A. I see no reason why it cannot be done.

Q. How could you positively distinguish an artery from a vein?

A. In brief, by their position, the thickness of their walls, and in the smaller arteries by their accompanying veins.

Q. What organ of the body has a complete circulation of its own, and to which of the three circulations does it belong?

A. Almost any organ may be said to have a circulation of its own, but the liver is probably meant here, and if so, it belongs to the portal circulation.

Q. What veins compose the portal circulation?

A. The mesenteric, gastric and splenic veins unite behind the head of the pancreas to form the portal vein. The portal vein is about four inches long; it enters the transverse fissure of the liver and divides into branches, which accompany the ramifications of the hepatic artery through the substance of the liver. The hepatic veins receive the blood and return it to the inferior vena cava.

Q. Is it possible to obtain an arterial circulation by injecting fluid into the right auricle of the heart?

A. Yes, it is possible, but not expedient or advisable, as the fluid must be forced through the pulmonary circulation to the left ventricle of the heart, then through the semilunar valves to the great aorta, which is not always possible, and when it is accomplished is certainly no improvement over the old method of injecting an artery.

Q. Give your reasons why a body should be embalmed either quickly or slowly.

A. Presuming that arterial embalming is meant, it should certainly be done very slowly to insure good results. From fifteen to twenty minutes time should be taken for every quart of fluid injected. The reason is obvious; when fluid is injected rapidly it soon fills all of the branches and sub-branches of the aorta, and if pushed rapidly onward some of the smaller vessels may rupture and cause serious leakage, but even if this does not occur the fluid is forced too rapidly into the tissues, often rupturing the capillaries, and allowing the fluid to escape from these little vessels, causing spots and mottling the skin; also, the fluid is not given a chance to become absorbed by the tissue, but is forced through the capillaries to the veins, and by increasing the quantity of the blood in those vessels it is often forced upwards to the face, causing serious discolorations.

Q. Which is the most important part of the body for the embalmer to understand?

A. The vascular system; but if an embalmer takes a proper interest in his profession, he will not be satisfied until he has a good knowledge of the general anatomy of the whole body. Let it be remembered that general does not mean surgical anatomy.

Q. Locate the arteries used in embalming and give the names of their accompanying veins.

A. The brachial artery is in the upper arm, and the accompanying veins are known by the same name; the radial is in the forearm, and the accompanying veins are called venae comites, or sometimes the deep radial veins; the common carotid is in the neck, and the accompanying vein is the internal jugular; the femoral is in the thigh, and the accompanying vein is known by the same name.

Q. How would you embalm a body to be shipped from Ohio to California in the month of July?

A. The weather being warm and the shipping point at a long distance, every precaution should be taken to insure success. Do arterial, cavity and needle work, inject the lumbar portions of the body hypodermically, pack all orifices with cotton and above all use a safe and reliable fluid.

Q. How young a child would you advise embalming arterially?

A. If the body was to be kept for a long time, I would advise embalming an infant arterially, but for the ordinary length of time the body of any child under five or eight years of age had best be treated by needle and cavity embalming.

Q. Should the head and shoulders of a body be elevated before or after embalming?

A. The head and shoulders should be elevated before embalming, to allow the blood to gravitate to the lower portions of the body, but when this is accomplished the body should be placed almost horizontally until the first three pints of fluid have been injected, provided always that no discolorations appear during the operation to indicate that the blood is being forced to the face, in which case, it should be immediately raised. After the first three pints of fluid have been injected, raise the body gradually as you continue to inject until the work is finished. This will insure an injection of the face and guard against discolorations, as there is little danger of flushing during the injection of the first three pints of fluid, and after that the fluid is forced rapidly into the veins, and by enlarging the quantity of liquid in them may cause it to flow into the face and give an undesirable color. If the capillaries of the face have already been injected these vessels will be constricted, leaving less room for the blood, and good results will follow. Whenever discolorations appear during injection, the blood should be drawn immediately, for while many fluids will bleach the blood, any of them are almost certain to leave an undesirable color.

Q. If on injecting the body one side of the face is found to be bleached and the other not, what is the cause and what would you do to remedy it?

A. Uneven circulation. Take up the artery on the unbleached side and carefully inject a small quantity of fluid.

Q. After a body had apparently been properly embalmed and been kept for three days, one of the arms turned green and gave forth an odor. What was the cause? What should be done?

A. Lack of collateral circulation in the arm. Take up the axillary artery and inject toward the distal end.

Q. Is the so-called arterio venous process of embalming practicable?

A. No; this so-called process requires the simultaneous injection of the brachial artery and basilic vein; should the first-named vessel happen to be obstructed by a thrombus, or in some other manner the results would be disastrous, for in that case the operator would be injecting the basilic vein alone. I see no advantage in its use.

Q. How much time is required for injecting a body arterially?

A. At least fifteen minutes for every quart of fluid injected.

Q. What would you do if you failed in your first attempt to secure good circulation of fluid through the arteries of a body that must be kept fifteen days?

A. Try again with another and larger artery. Failing, try to inject the body in sections, and whether successful or not inject by the needle process, fill the cavities, thoroughly inject the trunk of the body hypodermically and fill the air cells of the lungs.

Q. What diseases may you meet with that render arterial embalming very difficult if not impossible?

A. I know of no such diseases. In mutilated cases and floaters arterial embalming is sometimes impossible, but these are not diseases. The blood might, however, coagulate in the arteries in any disease, making it difficult or impossible to obtain an arterial circulation, but it would seldom happen.

Q. Could you secure a thorough circulation of fluid through a body even though the fluid did not pass through the lungs?

A. Yes. A thorough circulation in all other parts is possible even though the lungs may not be injected.

Q. While injecting the radial artery the skin often takes on a leathery appearance and exhibits other evidences of too much fluid in the forearm. What is the cause?

A. The radial artery is the smaller division of the brachial, and is often used by embalmers on account of its being very superficial and easily secured. It has twelve branches; the ulnar, the other division of the brachial, has ten. Whenever the fluid meets with any resistance in passing through the brachial artery, it seeks a course of less resistance and passes back through the ulnar, then through the palmar arch to the radial again, and, on account of the numerous branches which the two vessels possess, a large quantity of fluid is distributed to the tissues. When using this artery hold the hand up, or what is better tie it to something that will hold it in a perpendicular position, and allow the fluid to enter by gravitation. This will remedy the trouble spoken of.

Q. Does fluid enter the veins from the capillaries at any time?

A. Always when injected arterially.

Q. Does fluid injected into the arteries of a body as it leaves those vessels enter the veins and impregnate the blood therein contained?

A. The fluid injected into the arteries passes through the capillaries into the veins, and if it is a disinfectant will sterilize the blood contained in those vessels. The word impregnate, as used in the question, is badly chosen.

Q. How do you wash out the arterial system?

A. By raising and placing a drainage tube in the femoral artery, then injecting from the brachial or common carotid and forcing out the blood.

Q. What is the most important part of the body for the embalmer to understand?

A. He should be acquainted with all parts, but particularly with the vascular system.

Q. On which side of the heart do the arteries originate?

A. Systemic arteries on the left and the pulmonary on the right. Where the question is not qualified as above, I would say from both ventricles of the heart.

Q. How do you preserve the face?

A. When necessary, by injecting through the common carotid arteries.

Q. What is collateral circulation?

A. An indirect circulation through the connecting branches of an artery. Should the main branches be closed by a thrombus, collateral circulation may be obtained through one or more of the anastomosing arteries.

Q. How does the disease known as arteritis affect the vessels?

A. Dr. Roberts describes the first appearance of this disease as slightly raised patches on the lining membrane of the arteries, which, examined by a microscope, show a multiplication of the cells of the superficial layers of the inner coat of the vessels, thus leading to diminution of their calibre, to thrombosis, and in some cases to an arrest of the circulation. In cases of syphilis he says it is very liable to attack the vessels of the brain, thus stopping or greatly impeding the circulation in that organ. He cites several cases in which the larger arteries had become so thickened and obstructed as to make impossible the passage of the circulating fluid.

Q. In what cases is blood most likely to be found in the arteries?

A. My experience has taught me to look for blood in the arteries in all asphyxiated cases, and, in cases of sudden death by heart trouble or accidents where no arteries are severed, as in electric shocks.

Q. Does mutilation of the lungs interfere with arterial embalming and if so, why?

A. Yes, by allowing the fluid to escape from the mutilated vessel.

Q. How should you treat such cases?

A. That would depend upon the nature of the mutilation and many other conditions. If stabbed or shot through the lungs so as to cause the fluid to flow into the pleural cavities, the body must be opened and the arteries properly ligatured to obtain a complete circulation, but this is seldom necessary as the extremities can be injected in sections, the trunk of the body hypodermically, and with cavity embalming properly done, it can be kept in good condition indefinitely,

Needle Embalming

Q. What is meant by the so-called needle process of embalming?

A. The injection of the sinuses of the dura mater. Through these and the cerebral veins the brain is injected and preserved, after which a part of the fluid passes out through the spinal veins, but the largest part finds its way through the internal jugular veins to the innominate, and through those vessels to the superior vena cava, thence to the right auricle of the heart.

Q. If the injection is continued where will the fluid go?

A. It may take the course of the pulmonary circulation and find its way into the arteries, but will be more likely to pass into the inferior vena cava and thence through all of the veins, having no valves to stop its flow.

Q. How many so-called needle processes have been taught?

A. Four — the eye process, the Barnes needle process, the Champion needle process and the Dodge nasal process.

Q. Who were the first to teach each of these so-called processes of embalming?

A. To the best of my knowledge, F. A. Sullivan was the first man to teach the eye process. It has been said that it was first taught by Dr. Richardson of England, which may or may not be true; I do not know. The Champion needle process was first taught by Dr. Eliab Myers of Springfield, Ohio. The Barnes needle process was undoubtedly first taught by Dr. Carl L. Barnes, and the nasal process by the writer. Certain persons have lately learned (or say they have) that the so-called nasal process was discovered by one Rogers, but who Mr. Rogers was or where he belonged they do not say. It may be true that a man by that name first practised this method, but if so it is strange that after this method was known, so many much less convenient ones were studied out by such eminent men.

Q. Is it often necessary to use any of the so-called needle processes of embalming?

A. No; needle embalming should be used as an expedient only.

Q. In what cases should it be resorted to?

A. In cases of cerebral softening or hemorrhage, in cases of hydrocephalus (dropsy of the brain) and in all cases when for any reason arterial embalming has not been done.

Q. Can arterial embalming be done in this way?

A. As already stated, the fluid may take the course of the pulmonary circulation and pass from the right auricle through the tricuspid valves to the right ventricle, then through the semilunar pulmonary valves and along the pulmonary arteries to the lungs, thence through the pulmonary veins to the left auricle and from that chamber through the mitral valves to the left ventricle, then through the semilunar aortic valves into the arterial system; but as this will not always occur, it is not to be depended upon as a means of preserving a body.

Q. Describe the eye process?

A. When this process is attempted, the body should be placed on an incline. A needle is inserted at the inner corner of either eye, pushing it downward through the sphenoidal fissure, piercing the brain and reaching the confluence of the sinuses, or the torcular Herophili. From this point all of the sinuses of the dura mater receive the fluid, and through the cerebral veins, which open into these vessels, and have no valves, the brain is injected, and the fluid passes into the circulation as already described.

Q. What is the Barnes needle process?

A. A small six inch trocar is inserted at the back of the neck and passed through the foramen magnum, the great opening at the base of the skull, into the cavity of the cranium. The fluid is then injected and finds its way into the sinuses of the dura mater and, after the brain is filled, passes put through the internal jugular and spinal veins, as in all of the other processes and with the same results.

Q. What is the Champion process?

A. Drilling a hole, midway between the parietal bones of the skull, inserting a small trocar and injecting fluid. Fluid injected in this way would flow through the same vessels and accomplish the same purpose, as it would if injected by any other method; but it is very inconvenient, as well as unprofessional, to carry a bit and brace, and serious objections might be raised by the friends.

Q. What is the Dodge nasal process?

A. A small perforated needle, with diamond point, is inserted in either of the nostrils and easily pushed up through the cribriform plate of the ethmoid bone; the instrument is passed between the hemispheres of the brain to the superior longitudinal sinus, and by injecting the same results are obtained as by any of the other needle processes.

Q. What are the advantages of this process over all others?

A. The work is easily accomplished with absolutely no mutilation; there is no danger of bulging or discoloring the eye, as in the eye process; the bit or brace is not needed, as in the Champion process; it is much more easily accomplished than by the Barnes' method, and there is no leakage, as there always is when the needle is inserted through the opening at the base of the skull.

Q. In order to do needle embalming intelligently, with what vessels is it necessary to be acquainted?

A. With the sinuses of the dura mater and the other cerebral vessels.

Q. What are the sinuses of the dura mater?

A. Venous channels, differing from veins in that they have two coats, while veins have three.

Q. Are the sinuses of the dura mater of interest to embalmers? Give the number and names of those which terminate in the torcular Herophili.

A. Yes, the sinuses of the dura mater terminating in the torcular Herophili (a deep groove in the occipital bone, often called the wine press), are of much interest to the embalmer, on account of the necessity of his being acquainted with the so-called needle processes of embalming. They are six in number, and are called the superior longitudinal, the straight, the two lateral, and the occipital. Their outer coat is formed by the dura mater, and their inner coat by a continuation of the lining membrane of the veins.

Q. Describe the superior longitudinal sinus.

A. The superior longitudinal sinus begins in what is known as the foramen caecum, and runs over the central portion of the brain between the right and left hemispheres to the back of the skull, and terminates in the torcular Herophili.

Q. Describe the inferior longitudinal sinus.

A. The inferior longitudinal sinus, much smaller than the superior, commences at a point just below that vessel and, passing backward in the same manner, terminates in the straight sinus, which also enters into the torcular Herophili.

Q. Describe the lateral sinuses.

A. The lateral sinuses are of large size. They commence at the torcular Herophili and pass horizontally outward on either side of the head to the temporal bone, terminating in the internal jugular veins.

Q. Describe the occipital sinuses.

A. The occipital sinuses, two in number, commence in small veins, which communicate with the posterior veins, and terminate in the torcular Herophili.

Q. What is the function of the sinuses of the dura mater?

A. They receive the blood from the veins of the head and brain, and it is returned, largely through the internal jugulars, to the heart. These vessels, or channels, receive all of the cerebral veins.

Cavity Embalming

Q. What is cavity embalming?

A. The injection of the serous cavities of the body with disinfecting and preservative chemicals for the purpose of sterilizing and preserving the viscera therein contained.

Q. Describe the operation of cavity embalming.

A. Insert a trocar at a point about one and one-half inches below the point of the breast bone and in contact with the cartilage on the left side, attach an aspirator and remove any serum that may be present, then pass the instrument through the diaphragm and inject the pleural cavities, also the mediastinum and pericardium, and then, turning the trocar into the abdomen, fill that cavity with fluid. Puncture and inject the bowels, thereby sterilizing the alimentary canal, and your work by this method is complete. But in all cases where cavity embalming is to be depended upon to do the work, drawing the blood is to be recommended.

Q. Is there any other method of doing cavity embalming?

A. Yes, by combining needle and cavity work good results may be obtained with little or no mutilation. Insert the instrument, called the Dodge Cranium needle, in either of the nostrils, push it upward and into the cavity of the cranium, and inject as much fluid as possible. From one to three pints can easily be injected. Then fill the air cells of the lungs by using the trachea needle or lung trocar. This instrument can then be removed from the trachea and through the same aperture be passed beneath the clavicle and into the pleural cavities, and these spaces injected. The instrument can then be inserted under the umbilicus or navel and the abdominal cavity injected without apparent mutilation. This is a neat and effective way of doing cavity work, and is especially to be recommended when the friends insist on remaining in the room and seeing the work done. In giving these directions I have assumed that no arterial work is to be done.

Q. Can a body be preserved and thoroughly disinfected by cavity injection only?

A. Certainly not.

Q. in cavity embalming, state the organs and cavities which you think it necessary to inject.

A. The abdominal and each separate division of the thoracic cavity, namely, the pleural and mediastinal cavities. The organs cannot be injected by cavity embalming; they can only be surrounded by fluid.

Q. What precaution do you take in injecting the thoracic and abdominal, cavities to avoid puncturing arteries and destroying the circulation?

A. If arterial embalming has not been done I insert my trocar at a point about one and one-half inches below the point of the breast bone and pass it upward into the pleural cavities, keeping close to the ribs in order to avoid puncturing the lungs; then, keeping close to the breast bone to avoid the heart, I inject the mediastinal cavity. Withdrawing the instrument, I pass it downward into the abdominal cavity, keeping close to the abdominal wall to avoid puncturing the mesenteric and gastric arteries. After arterial embalming has been done and there is no reason to believe that there will be occasion for a second injection, no caution need be observed.

Q. Is it necessary to do cavity embalming in all cases?

A. No, cavity embalming is a supplementary measure. Six bodies out of every ten would keep as well if it were not resorted to.

Q. How many punctures are necessary in doing cavity embalming? Name the points of puncture.

A. It is seldom necessary to make more than one puncture for doing ordinary cavity work. The puncture should be made at a point one and one-half inches below and to the left of the breast bone, in contact with the costal cartilage.

Q. How do you inject the stomach and lungs?

A. The stomach with the trocar, or by use of the stomach tube. The lungs by the use of a curved needle inserted in the trachea.

Q. Can a body dead of dropsy be preserved by cavity embalming?

A. It is possible or even probable that a dropsical body might be preserved for a short time even though only cavity work were done, especially if the dropsical affection were confined to the cavities, and the liquid deposits had been drawn before the fluid had been injected. If the case were anasarca or tissue dropsy the chances of preservation would be very much diminished.

Q. Can an infant be successfully embalmed, if so, how?

103

A. Yes, by needle and cavity embalming. A small needle may be inserted through the nasal passage into the cranial cavity and a quantity of embalming fluid be injected. This, together with cavity embalming, is much better than arterial work, unless the body is to be kept for a long time. In this case the femoral or common carotid artery may be used, but the work must be done with great care.

Miscellaneous Questions Asked by State Boards

Q. What is rigor mortis? How soon after death does it set in?

A. Nervous contraction of the muscles and hardening of the muscle plasma or myosin, a colorless fluid peculiar to the muscles. It may come on in a few hours, as it usually does in bodies dying in perfect health, and may remain for an indefinite time, possibly for several days. It is longer delayed in emaciated bodies and disappears much sooner.

Q. What does flexibility following rigidity of the muscles indicate?

A. It indicates that rigor mortis has passed off, and it may be that putrefaction is at hand, but this is by no means certain. Many believe that no decomposition takes place while rigor mortis prevails, but it is an error. I have seen well-marked signs of putrefaction while the body was still rigid.

Q. On being called to a case we find a bad odor in the room and the body in a filthy condition, what is to be done?

A. Air the room, remove the filth, embalm and deodorize the body. We cannot always expect pleasant and agreeable conditions.

Q. How would you proceed to eliminate an offensive odor from a body apparently well preserved?

A. I would seek out the source from whence the odor was arising. When a body is apparently well preserved and there is a bad odor arising from it, the trouble is more than likely to be in the lungs or stomach, either arising from a gangrenous condition of the lungs or a cancerous condition of the stomach. If satisfied that it was from the lungs, I would inject the air cells of those organs through the trachea until the fluid appeared at the mouth, and then inject hypodermically over the chest walls a large quantity of fluid, to be absorbed through the intercostal spaces into the lungs. If the trouble was from the stomach, I would inject that organ with a good deodorizing fluid and if necessary withdraw the fluid and inject again.

Q. How would you proceed to restore a partially decomposed body?

A. By giving a thorough arterial and cavity injection, and if necessary resorting to hypodermic work. If not too badly decomposed, the body could probably be preserved and deodorized, but it is very doubtful if the features could ever be restored to their natural appearance, though they can often be greatly improved.

Q. What would you do if the embalmed body began to purge and mortify?

A. When a body begins to purge after being embalmed the supposition is that the work has not been properly done; I would, therefore, relieve the gas, and inject more fluid wherever I thought it was needed, thus expecting to arrest the further progress of putrefaction. I presume this is what is meant by the question, though the word mortify has a far different meaning from that evidently intended here.

Q. How would you supply every tissue of the body with fluid and not inject the cavities?

A. It might be impossible to do so, but it can usually be done by arterial embalming provided the vessels are free from thrombus or embolism.

Q. What conditions or cause of death will prevent complete circulation of the fluid, not including post mortems?

A. Aneurism of any of the large arteries; thrombus or embolism; arteritis or an atheromatous condition of the arteries may impede or hinder the circulation of the fluid. There are many mutilated cases in which it would be impossible to obtain a complete or even partial circulation.

Q. What is skin slip? Give the cause.

A. A slipping away of the epidermis or scarf skin from the true skin or derma. Its cause is decomposition; first of the areola tissue, which spreads to and involves the skin, causing softening of the rete mucosum, and allowing the covering to slip from its attachment. If the trouble is on the face, raise the carotid arteries and inject a fluid containing formaldehyde directly toward the head. The fluid injected in this way will be forced to the surface and prevent any further trouble. If on the hands, raise the axillary arteries and inject toward the distal end, and the result will be the same. If on the lower limbs, inject the femoral artery toward the feet. If on the unexposed parts of the body, inject hypodermically using a long trocar.

Q. How would you care for a body dead of lightning stroke?

A. I would embalm it as I would any other case as far as injecting arteries and cavities is concerned, taking care to ascertain if blood was present in the arteries. There is liable to be in these cases, and, if so, remove it. If there are burns on the exposed parts of the body use cosmetics to improve the appearance; the scars cannot be obliterated. A peculiarity of lightning stroke cases is that there is seldom any indication of rigor mortis.

Q. In injecting through the heart, which cavity would you use and why? How do you reach the cavity?

A. No well-informed and level-headed embalmer would ever inject a body through any of the chambers of the heart. Were he foolish enough to attempt it, the only chamber through which it would be possible to inject the arteries would be the left ventricle which can be reached by inserting a needle at a point about two and one-half inches to the left of the sternum, between the sixth and seventh ribs, pointing the trocar upwards and to the right; but such methods are only taught for advertising purposes, and would never be used even by those who teach them.

Q. What is the best method of injecting the lungs?

A. Use a small crooked instrument, called a trachea needle or lung trocar, insert it in the lower part of the trachea and push it downward; the air cells of both lungs can easily be injected in this way and show but little mutilation. A large crooked instrument is sometimes used and can be forced through the mouth and throat into the trachea, and the fluid injected; but the first-named method is the surest, quickest, neatest and best.

Q. What dangerous diseases do embalmers have to deal with that especially involve the alimentary canal?

A. Typhoid fever, Asiatic cholera, peritonitis and dysentery.

Q. In what division of the alimentary canal is gas usually found after death?

A. It may be found in any or all divisions, but most likely in the colon.

Q. What common chemical has a tendency to prevent coagulation of the bipod?

A. Sodium chloride (table salt).

Q. What is capillary congestion?

A. Large quantities of blood in the capillaries.

Q. In case of death from heart disease or an over dose of morphine is it possible for the arteries to be filled with blood, or for the veins to be emptied?

A. It is possible for the arteries to be filled with blood in bodies dead of any disease, but no more so in the case named than in any other. My experience has taught me to look for blood in the arteries in cases of asphyxiation, either by gas, drowning or strangulation. Veins are never empty unless the blood has escaped either by wounds before death or by removing it afterward.

Q. Name the orifices of the body.

A. Mouth, anterior nares (nostrils), anus, vagina.

Q. When bodies purge from what part of the body does the matter usually come?

A. Usually from the stomach; sometimes from the lungs.

Q. Is the spleen attached to the stomach?

A. The fold or section of peritoneum which invests the spleen and forms its outer or serous coat, is reflected on to the larger end of the stomach, but the organs are in no way attached one to the other.

Q. Where is the foramen magnum?

A. It is an aperture at the back of the head through the base of the skull communicating with the spinal canal, and through which the vertebral arteries enter the brain.

Q. In case of death during pregnancy would you treat the uterus by cavity injection; if so, at what point should the trocar be inserted?

A. Certainly; first pack the vagina, then insert the trocar at a point just above the pubic bone, push it inward and upward, piercing the womb, draw off the amniotic fluid, and inject embalming fluid. Treating a case of this kind in any other way is unsafe. Many embalmers and some teachers believe that the embalming fluid injected in the arteries of the mother finds its way to the foetus through the umbilical cord, but this is erroneous.

Q. After injecting is there danger of getting a bad color by drawing too much blood?

A. Drawing the blood does not always improve the color, but I think it seldom, if ever, makes it worse. If the face is too white the judicious use of a liquid face tint is advisable.

Q. What effect does heating the fluid have in arterial embalming?

A. When a formaldehyde fluid is used in concentrated form the use of warm water in certain cases is desirable, as it releases the gas and penetrates the body very rapidly. When fluid is used in the usual way heating is inconvenient and undesirable.

Q. What is meant by abdominal and pelvic post mortem?

A. An examination after death of the organic contents of these cavities.

Q. What is cranial evisceration?

A. The removal of the brain.

Q. What is meant by thoracic autopsy?

A. An examination for medical purposes of the viscera of the thorax.

Q. How do you remove discolorations when caused by a bruise?

A. Discolorations caused by a bruise cannot be wholly obliterated; a mixture of finely broken ice and salt applied like a poultice will sometimes cause improvement. A strong bleaching fluid injected hypodermically often helps much. Cosmetics may be finally applied.

Q. Does the urinary bladder ever cause trouble?

A. It may when filled, through fermentation of the urine.

Q. In case of death would you embalm a body at once?

A. It may be embalmed as soon as a permit from the coroner or a certificate from the attending physician can be obtained. Should signs of life or any suspicious circumstances about the case be noticed, I would report to the physician or coroner before embalming.

Q. Can you embalm a body from which all of the organs have been removed?

A. Partially or in sections by arterial injection. The trunk of the body can be preserved by cavity and hypodermic work.

Q. Are all dead bodies a menace to public health?

A. Not if properly cared for.

Q. What organ is the first to show putrefaction?

A. Usually, but not always, the intestines.

Q. What are proteids?

A. The albuminoid constituents of the body.

Q. What vessels are most likely to be affected by aneurism?

A. Any artery of the body may be affected in this way, but the ascending arch of the aorta is the most probable seat of the disease.

Q. What condition, if any, will require more than the average amount of fluid?

A. Any body in which putrefaction is already in an advanced stage, very large and fleshy bodies, especially dropsical cases, and bodies that are to be kept for a long time.

Q. Why do you get an ashy or putty color while using a formaldehyde fluid in arterial embalming?

Q. You get this phenomenon when the embalming fluid contains too much formaldehyde, and lacks the right quantity of other chemicals used to offset its effects. Chloride of zinc, a chemical used in some embalming fluids, is a frequent cause of the color complained of. This undesirable color is much more pronounced, however, in some cases than in others, owing to the chemical condition of the body produced by the disease or by the habits of the deceased during life.

Q. What is an anatomical stitch?

A. I know of no particular stitch called anatomical, but presume any stitch made on any part of the anatomy of the body might be called by that name. Smooth cuts on a dead body can be neatly closed by what is called the subcutaneous stitch, no thread being in sight except at the two ends of the wound.

Q. How should an ordinary case be shipped when the destination cannot be reached in thirty hours?

A. Presuming a non-contagious case is meant, consult rule 4 in the back part of this book. It is a part of the shipping rules that should be immediately changed.

Q. In case of death from diphtheria occurring in a room with other patients how would you proceed to take the body from the room, and place it in the casket and box to make it safe for the baggage-men to handle?

A. Convey the body to another room, not occupied by patients, embalm, disinfect and prepare as required by the rules of the health authorities.

Q. If called upon to prepare for burial a body dead of dropsy and the family insisted upon the remains being allowed to lie upon a couch in the parlor until after the funeral how would you proceed?

A. Remove the water from the body, embalm it and then comply with their wishes.

Q. What remedy can be used to prevent the skin on exposed parts of the body from drying up and turning brown? What is the cause of this phenomenon?

A. Dessication is best prevented by keeping the face or hands covered with a wet cloth or napkin. The New Century Bleacher is an excellent solution for this purpose, but clear cold water is much better than nothing. The chemicals contained in the fluid are the cause in many cases, at least the contributary cause, but it happens in very few bodies, proving the condition of the body to have more to do with it than the fluid. I have known it to happen in cases where no arterial embalming had been done.

Q. A body has been embalmed three days when large blisters appear on the lumbar portions. Give the cause. What is the remedy?

A. An escape of the watery portions of the body through the true skin, accumulating between that and the cuticle, forming blisters; cause unknown. Remove the blisters and inject a strong fluid hypodermically, using a trocar for this purpose.

Q. Can discolorations caused by jaundice be removed?

A. No, it is a stain; it can be helped by raising the carotid arteries and injecting a strong bleaching fluid into the face (it had better be a poisonous fluid) and then robbing magnesia into the skin with a piece of chamois. If the body is now placed beneath glass, or covered by a screen, the face will show a marked improvement.

Q. What organ is the last to show putrefaction?

A. That question cannot be answered, but in the absence of embalming I should say that organ which is composed of the most solid muscular tissues, perhaps the heart, or womb.

Q. What organ gives the embalmer the most trouble?

A. I know of no particular organ that gives the embalmer more trouble than any of the others; any diseased organ when attacked by bacteria may putrefy rapidly.

Q. How would you treat a child birth case where death was caused by hemorrhages before giving birth to the child?

A. By the usual method of arterial injection supplemented by washing out the uterus and packing with cotton.

Q. If the circulation were destroyed how would you fill the tissues with fluid?

A. If the circulation were completely destroyed, it would be impossible to wholly fill the tissues, but if it were only partially destroyed most of the tissues could be filled by injecting the body in sections. For instance, raise the common carotid arteries and inject the head, the axillary arteries and inject the arms, the iliac and inject the legs, then inject the air cells of the lungs through the trachea, fill the cavities and hypodermic the trunk of the body, and most of the tissues will be preserved.

Q. What causes swelling or puffing of the neck after drowning?

A. This phenomenon seldom occurs unless the body has been a long time in the water. When it does occur it is the result of decomposition of the subcutaneous tissue (beneath the skin), or is caused by water or gas in the lungs, which is very probable, as the apex of these organs extend above the collar bone to the roots of the neck.

Q. What is necessary to succeed in embalming at the present day?

A. A knowledge of general (not surgical) anatomy, of the physiology of the vascular system, at least a superficial knowledge of sanitary science, a chance to practise, and a cool head.

Q. Can a body dead of pneumonia be thoroughly embalmed?

A. The lungs are congested, but if fluid cannot be forced into them through the arteries, it can usually be accomplished by injecting the air cells through the trachea.

Q. If you were requested by the friends to use ice, instead of embalming, how would you proceed?

A. I would first try to convince them of the absurdity of so doing. If not successful and not provided with an icebox, I would place the body on the embalming board with a rubber blanket beneath it, put as large a cake of ice as possible in a pan and set it on the upper portion of the abdomen, place ice in pans at different points upon and around the body and cover the whole with another rubber blanket as tightly as possible; then have some one see to emptying the water as the ice melted and occasionally replenish it.

Q. Can a gaseous fluid be too strong for arterial work?

A. Yes. When a fluid contains more than 5 per cent formaldehyde gas it is liable to harden the body more than is desirable, and to give a bad color to the features. It must, however, contain that much in order to be antiseptic, unless other disinfecting chemicals are used.

Q. Would you embalm a body before there are some signs of decomposition?

A. Yes, unless there were reason to believe that life was not extinct.

Q. How should a case of death from child birth be treated?

A. The treatment would depend on the immediate cause of death. If from heart failure or excessive hemorrhage, which is frequently the cause, embalm in the usual way, after washing out and packing the vagina. If from puerperal fever treat as in any case of blood poisoning.

Q. Is it necessary to remove the brain or intestines in order to preserve a body?

A. Certainly not.

Q. How would you proceed to eliminate the offensive odor from a decomposing body?

A. I would embalm it thoroughly with a strong preservative, and make free use of a deodorizer.

Q. If called to a home where the family objected to embalming, what reason could you give in justification of the process?

A. I would try to impress them with the fact that embalming was much more effective, neater, and more humane than the use of ice. I would also try to convince them that I did but very little cutting and no mutilating, and if it were a contagious or infectious case I would explain the fact that the body could not be thoroughly disinfected in any other way.

Q. Give a good method for care of instruments after use.

A. Wash in a formaldehyde fluid for disinfection and polish with putz pomade.

Q. When you use the nasal tube how are you to know if the fluid enters the stomach or the air cells of the lungs?

A. You cannot tell as the contraction of the muscles after death may close the epiglottis or the slackening of the muscles may open it. The fluid is much more likely to find its way into the stomach than to the air cells of the lungs, but it frequently happens that the fluid will not pass to either place owing to the fact that both the epiglottis and the oesophagus are closed. It is much better never to use the nasal tube except for the purpose of washing out the nasal passage or mouth. When you wish to reach the air cells of the lungs insert a curved needle in the trachea and after elevating the body, inject, and the fluid will quickly pass to the lungs through the bronchial tubes. When you wish to enter the stomach do so with the trocar, which is easily accomplished, for when it is necessary to enter that organ it is always inflated with gas.

Q. What is the best method of injecting the stomach?

A. When the stomach is distended with gas, the neatest, quickest and best way is to insert a small trocar into the cardiac end of the stomach at a point reached by measuring one and one-half inches below the point of the breast bone and to the left until in contact with the cartilage or short ribs. Allow the gas to escape and then inject the fluid. If the stomach is not distended and rigor mortis has not set in, a stomach tube may be used, but is seldom necessary, for if there is no gas, no putrefaction is taking place, and after embalming will seldom occur.

Q. What causes gas to generate and what would you do to prevent it?

A. Gas is a product of the fermentative bacteria and when it appears it is simply an evidence of the change which is taking place, the natural process of the passing of the body into its original elements, "Ashes to ashes, dust to dust." It can be prevented by properly embalming the body before putrefactive changes have taken place.

Q. When the stomach and intestines are filled with gas, at what point would you puncture in order to allow it to escape?

A. At a point one and one-half inches below and to the left of the breast bone, in contact with the cartilage.

Q. Is there not danger of disturbing the circulation at this point?

A. No. When tapped at this point the instrument enters the large or splenic end of the stomach, and when that organ is distended, there is no danger of rupturing any large branch of the gastric or other arteries supplying the stomach.

Q. Is it necessary to puncture the intestines?

A. It often is, but it never should be done until the arterial work is finished, as the vessels are sure to be severed, thus preventing the circulation of the embalming fluid.

Q. In what part of the body do gases accumulate?

A. Gas may accumulate in almost any part of the body, but usually appears first in the large intestine.

Q. How is gas removed from the intestines?

111

A. If in the stomach or bowels, by puncturing those organs with the trocar, using the same aperture made for tapping the stomach. When the bowels are punctured, they should be kept from receding by placing the left hand on the lower portion of the abdomen and pressing upward. If gas accumulates in the pleural cavities, pierce the diaphragm from the same point at which you would puncture the stomach. If it accumulates in the air cells of the lungs, after the arterial work is done, pierce them by entering the trocar at a point midway between the breast bone and shoulder and between the second and third rib; or it maybe done from the same point as you would tap the stomach. Should gas accumulate in the areola tissue, insert the trocar beneath the skin and press it out.

Q. If called upon to embalm a very rigid body what would you do?

A. Flex the joints and break up the rigidity before embalming.

Q. In a body not embalmed, what does the disappearance of rigor mortis indicate?

A. That putrefaction will not be long delayed.

Q. How would you prepare a case of tuberculosis for shipment?

A. As provided in rule 3.

Q. In case of paralysis how do you preserve the paralyzed parts?

A. It is by no means certain that an arterial injection cannot be obtained in the paralyzed parts. They can usually be injected if sufficient pains be taken; however, should the injection be a failure, use a trocar beneath the skin and give a thorough hypodermic injection.

Q. What is the normal temperature of the living body? How high may the temperature be found after death?

A. The normal temperature of the living body is 98.1-2 degrees F. After death it usually falls, but may increase as high as 103 degrees F., and in very rare cases may be found even higher. However, this is of short duration; the temperature will soon fall to a point far below that of the living body.

Q. Why is the temperature of the dead body often very high?

A. The cause is not known. It is not a regular phenomenon and happens only in exceptional cases, and as far as my observation goes is not confined to any particular disease. Some claim that it may be expected in cases of tetanus, yellow fever, Asiatic cholera, electric shock, and intestinal diseases.

Q. How can you prevent mould?

A. Mould is the result of dampness; keep the body in a dry place. Some preparations for preventing mould have been compounded, but they are of doubtful value. It can usually be removed with alcohol.

Q. What is the advantage of being a licensed embalmer?

A. Only licensed embalmers are qualified to prepare bodies dead of certain diseases for interstate transportation, and they may prepare and ship certain other bodies without sealing the casket or bandaging the body. See Rules 2 and 3 of the shipping rules.

Q. What is always necessary in the treatment of a consumptive case?

A. It is always best to inject the air cells of the lungs and to tap the pleural cavities for serum, which they may or may not contain. Of course, it is always necessary to do arterial embalming.

SPECIAL CASES

Dropsy

Q. In a dropsical case where the whole body is involved, how would you proceed to remove the water and thoroughly supply every tissue with embalming fluid?

A. One way to remove water from the tissues, provided the operator is a skilled embalmer, is to raise a large artery, either the carotid or iliac, and its accompanying vein, and while injecting the artery draw blood and water from the tissues of the body through the vein. This can almost always be accomplished if the work is properly done. Another good method of removing water from the tissues is to pass a trocar beneath the skin of the lower limbs, making the insertion on either side of the ankle joint, and either side of the knee joint. By making several apertures the skin may be lifted from the flesh and the water given a chance to escape. Before performing this operation a rubber blanket should be placed over the embalming board and the sides rolled up in such a manner as to form a trough, the body be raised to a sharp incline, and a vessel placed at the end of the board to receive the water. The liquid will then gravitate to the dependent parts of the body and in a few hours' time large quantities will escape. If it is necessary to remove the water quickly, rubbing downwards with the hands or the application of a bandage will help to do so.

If only a small quantity of serum is present in the tissues it is not necessary to remove it; instead of doing so, raise the carotid arteries, tie one and placing an arterial tube in the other, inject towards the heart a fluid of double strength. The strength of a fluid can easily be doubled when using the concentrated Alcoform, by using two bottles to one-half gallon of water instead of one. When an ordinary fluid is being used strengthen it with formaldehyde, or chloride of zinc, or both, by adding about 6 per cent. When this solution is mingled with the serum it is diluted to the strength of an ordinary fluid and the body is safely embalmed, while if a fluid of the usual strength is used when mingled with the serous fluid of the body it becomes weakened and ceases to be a disinfectant, and the elements of putrefaction are not destroyed.

Q. How would you remove the water from the abdominal cavity?

A. First elevate the body as high as the. embalming board will allow, then insert the aspirating tube at a point just above the pubic bone and pass it into the pelvic cavity. The water will gravitate from the abdomen and be easily removed.

Q. How would you remove the water from the pleural cavities?

A. Using the same aperture made for tapping the stomach, I would pass the dropsical needle first into one and then into the other pleural cavity and use the aspirator.

Q. The hands are often found filled with water until they are abnormally large, how would you remove it and show no abrasions on the hands?

A. Using a small sized twelve inch trocar, insert it at a point about midway between the hand and elbow joint, and pass it under the skin to the hand several times, raising the integument from the flesh. Then by raising the hand high, the water can easily be removed by pressure.

Q. How would you treat a case of dropsy of the lower limbs?

A. If the tissues do not contain a large quantity of water, make the fluid of double strength, raise the external iliac arteries and inject at least a pint of fluid toward the distal end of each limb. If there is a large quantity of water in the tissues it should be removed.

Q. In a case, of hydrocephalus how do you remove water from the ventricles of the brain?

A. Using a small eight-inch trocar, pass the instrument into either of the anterior nares (nostrils) and press it upwards into the cranial cavity (as in the needle process) and the water will escape. After the water has been removed inject a few ounces of fluid and pack the nostrils with cotton.

Q. In a case of hydro-pericardium (dropsy of the heart) how would you remove the water?

A. Insert a needle at a point about two and one-half inches to the left of the sternum, between the fifth and sixth ribs, pushing the instrument a little to the right, and piercing the pericardium. If the sac is filled with water it will be an easy matter to attach an aspirator and remove it.

Q. In case of oedema of the lower limbs where a moderate quantity of water is present in the tissue, how could you treat it without removing the water?

A. Raise the femoral, or better, the iliac arteries, and using a very strong fluid, at least double its usual strength, inject towards the distal end from one pint to one quart in each limb; this will insure the preservation of the parts and save removing the water.

Q. If blisters form on any part of the trunk of the body how would you proceed to remove them and prevent any further formations of the same kind?

A. Break the blisters and remove the water and then the cuticle; then inject a good quantity of strong fluid hypodermically.

Q. What causes blisters to form?

A. It is an exudation of serum from the tissues of the body, which accumulates between the true skin and the cuticle. Just why this will happen in some bodies, while it does not in others, is a question which cannot be answered. It usually occurs in dropsical cases, but may happen in bodies dead of almost any disease.

Drowning

Q. How would you treat a case dead of drowning?

A. If there are no discolorations of the exposed parts, first attend to removing water from the lungs. This can be done by drawing the tongue out of the mouth as far as possible, placing the body on the chest with some kind of a block underneath it, and pressing between the shoulders, to force the water from the air cells of the lungs through the bronchial tubes and the trachea. This is almost always successful. Then raise an artery and inject the body. In this, as in all other asphyxiated cases, it is more than likely that blood will be found in the arteries. If so, it should be removed.

Q. How can this be accomplished?

A. By raising the femoral artery and inserting a large tube, attached to a rubber hose, the free end of which is lead into a fluid bottle, and injecting the artery you have raised for that purpose, which will force the blood from the arteries into the bottle. When the blood is washed out the fluid will appear clear or very nearly so. The femoral artery should then be tied and the injection continued.

Q. When death has been caused by drowning and the body has been in the water four or five days, how would you treat it?

A. The treatment would depend upon the season, and the condition of the body; if in an advanced state of decomposition it had best be buried as soon as possible; if not, relieve the gas, remove the water from the lungs, embalm arterially, fill the cavities, do thorough hypodermic work, and inject the air cells of the lungs. In this case always use a fluid of double strength on all parts except the face, which can be done by raising and tieing the carotid arteries, and injecting the face separately with a milder fluid.

Q. In cases dead of drowning when the neck begins to swell or puff up what do you do?

A. First ascertain the cause. If it is decomposition of the tissues, relieve the gas and inject hypodermically. If it is gas or possibly water in the lungs, remove it, and then inject the air cells of the lungs through the trachea.

Q. What is a floater?

A. A body that has been in the water for a certain period of time will come to the surface and remain there and is often called a floater.

Q. How should these cases be treated?

A. Unless the friends were willing to pay well for the trouble and expense necessary for the preservation of such a case, it should be buried at once, which is the most sensible thing to do.

Q. Can such a case be preserved and its natural appearance restored?

A. These cases can be preserved for an indefinite period of time, but the natural appearance cannot be restored.

Q. What is it necessary to do in order to preserve such a case?

A. Wash the body thoroughly. Then release the gas from the cavities and inject a strong fluid, taking care not to rupture the circulation while so doing.

Do not inhale the escaping gas, but allow it to pass into the open air if possible through a long rubber hose. After this is done raise an artery and inject as much fluid as the body will receive, using chemicals of double strength. When this is absorbed release the gas from the subcutaneous tissue by thrusting the trocar beneath the skin and pressing the gas out, allowing it to escape through a long rubber tube, the free end of which has been placed in a bottle of fluid. Having removed as much gas in this way as possible, inject a large quantity of fluid hypodermically. The fluid injected should contain at least double the usual quantity of chemicals: Should this fail to accomplish the desired results, pack the body in a mixture of sawdust and hardening compound, using at least five packages of compound with a sufficient quantity of dry sawdust to completely cover the body. For this purpose use a rough box, make a layer of compound and sawdust on the bottom of the box, lay the body on this and completely cover it, allow it to remain from forty-eight to seventy hours when it will be found to be hard and odorless.

Tumors

Q. What are tumors?

A. Tumors are abnormal growths that are liable to appear in any part of the body. Some are malignant, others are not.

Q. What tumors are most likely to give the embalmer trouble?

A. Ovarian tumors, which are attached to the ovaries in women. They are of three kinds, cystic, cellular and hard or fibrous tumors.

Q. Describe the different kinds.

A. A cystic or hollow tumor is a sac containing more or less fluid. A cellular or mixed tumor is full of cells, which are filled with water. A hard tumor appears to be a mass of fibrous and fatty tissue. The last named will give the embalmer little or no trouble. It is only necessary to remove the water which surrounds it, and inject a small quantity of fluid into the pelvic cavity.

Q. How should tumors of the other varieties be treated?

A. If it is a cystic tumor, insert an aspirating tube and remove the water, after which inject a small quantity of embalming fluid. If a cellular tumor, break down the cells by inserting the trocar many times; then withdraw all the water possible and after that is accomplished inject preservatives. In all cases of ovarian tumors, ascities or peritoneal dropsy may be expected, and care should be taken to remove all the water possible and inject fluid in its place.

Cancers

Q. What treatment should be given bodies dead of cancer?

A. A malignant tumor or cancer is a growth of great variety, the most common being the epithelioma or epithelial cancer. This variety starts in the skin, the usual seat of the disease being the lip, corner of the eye or inside the nostril. When death ensues from a cancer of this nature it often happens that the sore has eaten into the tissues of the face leaving it unsightly. The best treatment is to wash the part with a strong fluid and then fill it with hardening compound, covering this with a bandage and letting it remain until the diseased tissues are hardened and deoderized, and then brush out the compound and fill the aperture with plaster of paris. Make the surface perfectly smooth, and when hard, tint it as near flesh color as possible. Apply it to any other parts of the face the case may suggest in order to get the best effect possible. In this way bodies that would otherwise have presented a disgusting appearance may be made to look quite well. Cancers of the breast, or any unexposed part of the body, may be treated with applications of hardening compound and bandaged.

Q. When there is but one cancer visible is there liable to be more in the interior of the body?

A. Yes, bodies dead of this disease, have been found to have cancers in different parts of the body; therefore, in cases of this kind every precaution must be taken to insure success by supplementing the arterial embalming with thorough cavity and needle work.

Aneurism

Q. What is an aneurism?

A. A cystic tumor consisting of a dilated artery or communicating with the canal of the vessel and formed by its walls, which become dilated to a large extent and often ruptures. When the aneurism is located on the ascending arch of the aorta, which is the most frequent seat of the disease, and all of its walls ruptured, death is the result.

Q. Can a body dead of this disease be embalmed arterially without tieing the ruptured vessel?

A. No. The fluid would escape through the opening in the arterial wall.

Q. How would you proceed to embalm a body dead of aneurism in the arch of the aorta.

A. If necessary to hold the body for a long time, the thorax may be opened and the tumor removed, after which the vessel should be properly ligatured, and then the embalming may be proceeded with. This, however, is an operation that requires skill, and one to which the friends would probably object, and it is not advisable for the embalmer to attempt it unless he has the consent of the family, and the assistance of the attending physician. Otherwise he had best inject the body in sections and do cavity and needle work, which if skillfully accomplished will hold a body for an indefinite period of time.

Q. What do you mean by injecting in sections?

A. Raise the common carotid artery and inject, toward the face, about one-half pint of fluid. This must be done slowly and carefully. Then raise the axillary arteries and inject toward the distal end of the arm. This will preserve the upper extremities. Now raise the iliac or femoral arteries and inject the legs, and all except the trunk of the body has been injected, which can be taken care of by cavity and hypodermic work done as directed in another part of this work.

Gangrene

Q. What is gangrene?

A. The death of a certain part of a body while the main portion lives is called gangrene or mortification. Usually the immediate cause of this disease is the obstruction of an artery, but this seldom occurs in a healthy person. Those who die of gangrene are usually persons who have long been affected with diabetes, Bright's disease of the kidneys, or some other chronic complaint of long standing. This disorder may manifest itself in many forms; what is called dry gangrene, when the parts become black and dry, and what is known as moist or putrefactive gangrene , are the most common.

Q. How would you treat a case of this kind?

A. If the parts affected are the outer portion of a body such as a foot or limb, bandage in hardening compound. This will arrest the progress of putrefaction and destroy all odor. Should the trouble be mortification of the bowels, these organs should be punctured and a strong deodorizing and disinfecting fluid injected, after which a sufficient quantity must be injected into the cavity to cover the viscera. This should never be done, however, until the arterial injection has been accomplished. Gangrene sometimes attacks the lungs in cases of consumption, owing to an insufficient arterial supply. This will be made manifest by an odor arising from the body, when it is apparently well preserved. Should this happen, inject the air cells of the lungs thoroughly and give a good hypodermic injection over the walls of the chest, as the lungs are probably adhered to the walls of the thorax and the fluid thus injected will find its way into the lungs by penetrating its walls.

Alcoholism

Q. Describe the anatomical conditions of a body dead of alcoholism?

A. Catarrh of the stomach and often ulceration of that organ, together with enlargement of the liver, and a flabby degenerated heart, are some of the conditions found in bodies dead of this affection. The arteries will either be found hardened or peculiarly softed and sometimes obstructed. The kidneys are usually very much affected, often causing a more or less dropsical condition of the abdominal cavity. Capillary congestion is liable to be a condition which may cause embarrassment to the embalmer, and the cerebral vessels may be diseased, preventing a circulation in the brain.

Q. After arterial embalming, what measures are necessary to insure success in caring for a body dead of this affection?

A. As a thrombus is liable to obstruct the arterial circulation and as these cases are liable to decompose rapidly when not thoroughly injected, every precaution should be taken. The blood should always be withdrawn and any serous fluid found in the cavities removed. Embalming arterially should be supplemented by cavity and needle work. Owing to the abnormal chemical conditions spots are liable to appear on the face. To prevent this keep that portion of the body covered with a napkin which has been saturated with a good bleaching and preserving fluid. Bodies dead of this disorder should be closely watched as putrefaction of the fatty tissues may occur at any time. Should this be noticed it should be arrested at once by the use of the hypodermic needle.

Erysipelas

Q. Is erysipelas a difficult case to preserve, and if so, why?

A. Yes. Erysipelas is characterized by inflammation of the skin, also involving the subcutaneous and in some cases the muscular tissues. Pus is often found under the cuticle, or in the cellular tissue beneath the skin, and the disease frequently terminates in gangrene. The superficial veins are almost always found congested, causing serious discolorations to appear, and owing to the abundance of putrefactive bacteria, which are always present, decomposition of bodies dead of this disease is usually rapid.

Q. What should be done to arrest the progress of putrefaction?

A. Embalm the body in the usual way, injecting more than the average quantity through the arteries. As pus is very likely to form in the areolar tissue beneath the skin, putrefaction is liable to take place there and progress rapidly. This can be arrested by injecting fluid hypodermically. As the blood is dark in color and very liable to stain the skin, should it find its way to the exposed parts, it is advisable to remove it. Care should be exercised in treating bodies dead of this disease, for should there be abrasions on the hands it is very easy to become affected by the germs gaining entrance to the circulation, and as it is claimed by some that persons have been infected where no wounds or abrasions of any kind existed, the use of gloves is to be recommended.

Septicemia

Q. What is the meaning of the terms septicemia and pyemia?

A. Blood poisoning. The two terms have almost the same meaning, pyemia being only a secondary condition.

Q. Are bodies dead of blood poisoning hard to preserve or dangerous to handle?

A. Yes; both. However, if the embalming is properly done and due care used in handling, there is little danger of losing the body or of infection to the embalmer.

Q. How would you treat a case of septicemia in order to insure success?

A. Withdraw all of the blood that can be removed. Aspirate all the bloody serum from the serous cavities, and give a thorough arterial injection, as in these cases both the blood and tissues appear to contain immense quantities of putrefactive bacteria. If there is slipping of the epidermis, which there is liable to be, inject fluid beneath the skin, provided the part affected is unexposed. If the face is affected, inject that part through the common carotid arteries. As discolorations are very liable to appear on the face of bodies dead of blood poisoning, an application of New Century Bleacher is advisable.

Syphilis

Q. Are syphilitic bodies dangerous to the embalmer?

A.. Not if due care is used in handling. The greatest danger lies in the fact that we seldom know when we are treating them, as the cause of death is seldom given. In operating upon a body where the disease is known, the embalmer should either wear rubber gloves or take the precaution to rub his hands thoroughly with an antiseptic grease; vaseline well charged with carbolic acid is an excellent thing to use. He should be careful not to cut or prick himself with an instrument that has been used on a body of this kind, as inoculation with the poison of the disease might be the result.

Q. Is any special treatment necessary in this disease?

A. In chronic cases of syphilis the arterioles and capillaries are liable to become constricted to such a degree, as to make it doubtful if a thorough injection of the vascular system can be obtained, and as the cerebral vessels are most likely to be affected in this way, a resort to the needle process as a supplementary measure after the arterial work has been done is advisable. This will take care of the brain and give a partial venous circulation, which if not strictly necessary is certainly desirable.

Peritonitis

Q. What is peritonitis?

A. It is an inflammation of the serous membrane which lines the posterior walls of the abdomen and invests the viscera in the abdominal cavity. It may arise from various causes. The most frequent is a strain, a blow on the abdomen or a penetrating wound, but certain forms of the disease are believed to be caused by a germ.

Q. What are the anatomical conditions of a body dead of peritonitis?

A. The abdominal viscera will be found in a highly inflamed condition, with the liver and spleen usually enlarged. Large quantities of serous deposits are often found in the peritoneal cavity, sometimes mixed with blood and pus, and often of a thick greasy nature. These deposits are often coagulahle and occasionally purulent.

Q. How should a body dead of this disease be treated in order to insure success?

A. After the arterial embalming has been done the attention of the operator should be turned to the abdominal cavity. If a large amount of gas is found in the intestines it should be removed by tapping the stomach and pressing on the lower portion of the abdomen. When this is accomplished, inject from one to two quarts of fluid diluted with water into the abdominal cavity, and then knead the bowels, thereby dissolving and diluting the serous deposits so that it may be removed with the aspirator. The body should then be elevated as high as the embalming board will allow and an aspirating tube inserted in the pelvis, making the aperture just below the pubic bone, the aspirator attached and the deposit removed. A very strong fluid should then be injected into the abdominal cavity, in sufficient quantity to cover the viscera; the bowels should be punctured and fluid freely injected into these organs; all orifices of the body should then be packed with cotton, after which the work of embalming is complete, and the body should keep for an indefinite period of time.

Cerebral Hemorrhage

Q. What causes cerebral hemorrhage?

A. Calcification or degeneration of the vessels of the brain. Any excitement or emotion, or sudden or vigorous exertion, may be the immediate cause of the rupture or giving way of the cerebral vessels.

Q. What special treatment should be given to a body dead of this disease?

A. As the rupture of the cerebral vessels is usually the result of congestion, after arterial embalming has been done, an injection by the nasal process is advisable. This will force the blood from the sinuses of the dura mater and relieve the venous congestion, which if not relieved, may cause serious discoloration of the face. While the fluid is being injected by the needle process, draw the blood, thus creating a vacuum in the great deep veins and making it much easier to relieve the congestion in the upper portions of the body.

Cerebral Softening

Q. Give a description of cerebral softening, commonly called softening of the brain, and state how bodies dead of this disease should be treated.

A. Cerebral softening, or softening of the brain, is most frequently the result of a diseased condition of the walls of the small arteries and capillaries, which constrict these vessels, causing an insufficient blood supply and constant lack of nourishment to the tissue of the brain, which become softened, in some cases almost to the condition of a fluid pulp. In addition to arterial embalming at least a pint of fluid should be injected into the substance of the brain by the Dodge nasal process. If this is done in season no trouble will ensue, but when neglected the brain has been known to decompose rapidly, causing the eyes to bulge and matter to escape from the ears and even appear at the corner of the eyes. This is caused by gas generated from a putrefying brain, and unless the trouble is remedied at once failure will be the result. Should this happen, the embalmer should introduce an eight-inch trocar through the nasal passage into the brain. The result will be the escape of a quantity of semi-fluid matter mixed with blood. Allow this to escape, and inject fluid through the same instrument into the brain, lowering the head in order to saturate the brain thoroughly; then pack the aperture tightly with cotton and no further trouble need be apprehended.

Typhoid Fever

Q. What parts of the body are affected when death is the result of typhoid fever?

A. The liver, spleen, and kidneys, and sometimes the thoracic viscera are inflamed, but the large and small intestines are the parts most affected.

Q. Aside from an arterial injection what treatment would you give a body dead of this disease in order to insure its preservation?

A. First remove the gas, and any serous matter that may be found in the abdominal cavity, then puncture and inject the bowels with a sufficient quantity of fluid to thoroughly sterilize the alimentary canal. Inject a sufficient quantity of fluid into the abdominal cavity to cover the viscera. When necessary draw the blood. In this, as in all cases, where the bowels are inflamed, the embalmer should not neglect to pack the apertures tightly with cotton.

Q. Describe minutely the course you would follow in removing gas from a body dead of typhoid fever?

A. Having done my arterial embalming and removed the serum from the abdominal cavities, I would attach a rubber hose to my trocar and lead the free end of it into a bottle of fluid, then puncture the stomach and bowels, allowing the gas to pass into the fluid. This would deodorize and disinfect it.

Consumption

Q. Does the fluid ever escape from the mouth or nostrils while injecting bodies dead of consumption?

A. Yes.

Q. What is the cause of this phenomenon?

A. A rupture of either the bronchial or pulmonary circulation which would allow the fluid to escape from these vessels and flow into the air cells of the lungs, from which it could easily pass into the bronchial tubes and thence through the trachea and out of the mouth or nostrils.

Q. What would you do in a case of this kind?

A. If the body is to be kept for a long time, make a leaflike incision in the skin just above the sternum or breast bone, raise the integument and uncover the trachea; then make a small incision in the trachea and fill it with cotton, and, using a full curved needle and a strong string, pass the needle under the trachea and tie that organ tightly; this will prevent any further escape of fluid.

Pneumonia

Q. Describe the morbid condition of a body dead of pneumonia?

A. Oedema of the lungs (water in the air cells) is liable to be a condition of this disease. The color of the lung tissue is a reddish brown, and when cut a bloody serum often escapes. In many cases serous fluid is found in the pleural cavities. The right chambers of the heart and great veins attached to the auricle are well filled with blood which is very liable to be coagulated.

Q. How would you treat a case of this kind?

A. If no discolorations on the exposed parts are noticed, first inject the body arterially, being careful to inject very slowly. This accomplished insert the aspirator tube and test the pleural cavities for serum; draw the blood when necessary by tapping the right auricle of the heart, or using the internal jugular vein, as in this case a small vessel will seldom answer the purpose on account of the tendency of the blood to coagulate.

Pletiritis

Q. What is pleuritis?

A. Inflammation of the pleura, more commonly called pleurisy.

Q. Should any special treatment be given a body dead of this disease?

A. The operator should be careful to draw the water from the pleural sacks, remove serous matter from the lungs and inject the air cells of those organs with fluid. In this disease a large quantity of fluid is sometimes found in one of the pleural cavities, which may push the heart to one side, making it difficult for the operator to reach the right auricle for the purpose of drawing blood.

Purpura

Q. Describe the disease known as purpura.

A. This disease is characterized by rupture of the capillaries and extravasations of blood in various parts of the body, causing spots to appear on the exposed surfaces, which are very difficult to treat successfully. If the spots are on the face, it is just possible to remove them by injecting that part through the common carotid artery. If this is not successful a hypodermic needle and a good bleaching fluid properly used will at least improve the appearance. Supplement this with cosmetics skillfully applied and a great improvement will be noticed. Cavity and needle work is always advisable in this disease as collateral circulation may not be obtained.

Paralysis

Q. Why should the embalmer not be able to secure a circulation in a body that has been paralyzed?

A. A certain portion of a living body may be partially paralyzed by a blood clot, which may be and usually is called an embolism; in that case the free flow of blood through the vessels in that part is impeded and the vessels become constricted. General paralysis is usually caused by an affection of the brain or spinal cord, and lack of motion in the voluntary muscles causes a shrinkage of all the organs including the blood vessels, and consequently the circulation of the fluid may be impeded, but it is seldom or never entirely obstructed.

Q. In case of paralysis how do you preserve the paralyzed parts?

A. It is by no means certain that an arterial injection cannot be obtained in the paralyzed parts. They can usually be injected if sufficient pains be taken; however, should the injection be a failure, use a trocar beneath the skin and give a thorough hypodermic injection.

Jaundice

Q. Can the color be improved in a yellow jaundice case? How would you treat it?

A. It is claimed by some authorities that the discoloration in this disease is due to rapid absorption of the bile, after its formation, by the veins and lymphatics, while others claim that it is due to lack of secretion by the liver and consequent retention of the bile and pigment in the blood. My opinion is that the last is the correct version, but, however that may be, it is certain that the skin is stained as though it were done by dyeing and the embalmer should not be expected to remove it. These cases can, however, be made to look much better by the judicious use of fluids and cosmetics. Inject directly to the face through the common carotid artery a strong bleaching fluid, then inject the body, after which depend on the use of a cosmetic to take care of the face and other exposed parts, brighten the skin with face tints and then, using a chamois skin and magnesia, rub the powder on the face and a marked improvement will be noticed. Formaldehyde fluid should never be used for the purpose of injecting the face as it is very liable to turn it green. A fluid composed largely of arsenic and chloride of zinc is the best for this purpose.

Mother with Child

Q. When injecting the body of a pregnant woman, does the fluid injected into the arteries of the mother reach the foetus and inject it also?

A. I am of the opinion that it does not.

Q. What treatment should be given a body of this kind?

A. After arterial embalming has been done, a trocar should be inserted at a point just above the pubic bone and pushed upward and backward to pierce the womb and draw away the amniotic fluid; then embalming fluid should be injected to preserve the foetus.

Sunstroke

Q. How should a body dead of sunstroke be treated?

A. Sunstroke or insolation is a term used to signify a collapse of the central nervous system caused by extreme heat and its effect upon certain organs of the body. The principal changes in the body after death from heat stroke are anaemia of the brain and congestion of the lungs, together with softness of the heart and the muscular tissues generally. The blood will be found in a liquid condition, but very dark. Give the body a thorough arterial injection and draw the blood, for should this liquid, being very dark, be forced to the exposed parts serious discolorations would result. It is often advisable to supplement this work by cavity and needle embalming, as it is always very warm weather when we have such cases.

Electric Shock

Q. What unusual morbid conditions, if any, are peculiar to bodies dead of an electric shock?

A. As the central nervous system is instantly paralyzed, the muscular contraction of the walls of the arteries, by which the blood is forced out of those vessels, may not take place, therefore, the blood usually remains and should be removed before injecting. Usually very little rigor mortis is observed, although there are exceptions to this rule. If the body is not burned the treatment need not be different from ordinary cases.

Poisoning

Q. Is there any special treatment for a body, where death was due to poisoning?

A. It has often been asserted that cases of morphine poisoning are very difficult to embalm successfully, as putrefaction is rapid even after injection, but I have found no difficulty in preserving bodies dead from any form of poisoning, and know of no morbid conditions that will materially interfere with successful embalming.

Tuberculosis

Q. How would you treat a case dead of tuberculosis to insure its preservation for an indefinite period?

A. Embalm the body arterially and, after removing any serous deposits that may be found in the pleural or abdominal cavities, inject those spaces with fluid if it is deemed necessary, then inject the air cells of the lungs and in most cases this will complete the work.

Thrombus

Q. What is meant by a thrombus or embolism?

A. A thrombus or embolism is a somewhat common affection and consists in the stoppage of a vessel by a fibrinous plug, or by calcareous matter deposited by the blood.

Appendicitis

Q. What part of the alimentary canal is most affected in bodies dead of appendicitis.

A. The vermiform appendix, caecum and usually the large and small intestine, peritonitis is often a complication of this disease.

Swelling of the Neck

Q. What is the cause of the phenomenon known as swelling of the neck?

A. Putrefaction of the fatty tissues beneath the skin is the usual cause, but it may be the result of fermentation of the serum contained in the pleural cavities, the gases pressing upwards beneath the loose skin which covers the neck.

Q. How can the size of the neck be reduced?

A. Pass a trocar beneath the skin of the neck, making the insertion from some point where the mutilation will not show, remove the gas, and inject fluid hypodermically. The fluid will be quickly absorbed and prove a complete remedy. providing the trouble is in the tissues. Should it arise from serum in the pleural cavities, remove the serum and inject fluid into the pleural sacks.

Miscellaneous Questions

Q. Under what condition would you be most likely to contract the disease while handling a case of diphtheria or tuberculosis?

A. The condition of one's health would have much to do with it. A person having a tendency to consumption by reason of scrofulous or syphilitic affections or by inheritance should be careful of exposure, especially in unsanitary and badly ventilated rooms. Adults in good health will seldom contract diphtheria as it is a disease peculiar to children.

Q. When in doubt as to the nature of a case you may be handling, how would you treat it?

A. Embalm and disinfect it, taking care to do both in a thorough manner.

Q. What character or kinds of cases are most difficult to restore after putrefaction has commenced?

A. Those cases where a fermentative process has taken place in the blood causing capillary gas. These conditions are most likely to result from blood poisoning and puerperal fever cases.

Q. In what cases is death quickly followed by putrefactive changes?

A. Putrefaction is likely to take place quickly in bodies dead of alcoholism, septicemia, puerperal fever, erysipelas, dropsical cases, peritonitis, typhoid fever and uremic poisoning.

Q. Why are bodies dead of these diseases liable to decompose rapidly?

A. Owing to the morbid condition of the body and the multiplicity of the putrefactive germs.

Post Mortem and Mutilated Cases

Q. If the liver, stomach and spleen had been removed, what vessels would it be necessary to tie in order to inject the body arterially?

A. The hepatic, gastric and splenic arteries, which supply all of the organs named arise as terminating branches of the coeliac axis, a short, stout artery one-half inch in length, which originates in the aorta just below the diaphragm. I would find this vessel and place a ligature on it; when this has been done no fluid can escape.

Q. If the brain only were removed how would you proceed to embalm the body?

A. An attempt should be made to tie the internal carotid and vertebral arteries. If successful, embalming would be easy, but experience has shown that this is a hard task to perform; should you fail to accomplish it fill the cavity of the skull below the section with plaster of Paris, pressing it down into the carotid canal and the foramen magnum, the opening in the skull through which the internal carotid and vertebral arteries enter, and these vessels will probably be closed and no fluid escape while the body is being injected.

Q. How would you proceed if the kidneys had been removed?

A. Tie the renal arteries.

Q. If the bladder or womb had been removed what vessels must be tied before injecting?

A. The internal iliac arteries and veins. They will be found about two inches below the bifurcation of the abdominal aorta.

Q. How would you embalm a body from which the lower limbs had been severed?

A. I would ligature the severed arteries and veins and inject the body and the limbs separately; then join the parts together with splints and bandage them, placing hardening compound between the parts to prevent putrefaction.

Q. If, after the arteries had been tied and injection commenced, there were leakage through the collateral branches, how would you proceed?

A. Place a strong cord around the part, and, using a lever, twist the cord until very tight. This will prevent any considerable leakage.

Q. If all the viscera in the trunk of the body were removed, including the great aorta, would partial arterial embalming still be possible?

A. Yes; the body could be embalmed in sections, the head through the common carotid arteries, the arms through the axillary arteries, and the lower limbs through the iliac or femoral arteries.

Q. How would you preserve the viscera in a case of this kind?

A. The quickest, neatest and best way is to pack it in hardening compound, but a strong fluid can be used for the purpose. When fluid is used, it should be of double strength and a sufficient quantity used to cover the viscera completely. After this has been done cover the organs with a couple of layers of absorbent cotton to prevent leakage, and sew the body up, taking care to thoroughly saturate the severed parts with fluid, for if this is neglected and the weather is warm an odor may arise or the parts may become filled with maggots caused by flies.

Q. How would you treat the trunk of the body in order to insure its preservation?

A. It can be preserved by hypodermic injection.

Q. If the head were severed from the body by a mill or railroad accident how would you proceed to embalm and make the body presentable?

A. First inject the head through the common carotid arteries, then secure the same vessels in the trunk of the body; tie one and inject the other. Should the fluid quickly return through the veins tie those vessels. The head and body being now preserved, take a stiff stick, sharpen it at both ends and insert it in the trunk, then place the head on the other end of the stick, thus forming a false neck. Before joining the head to the trunk of the body saturate the raw flesh with fluid, or place hardening compound between the parts, and sew them together neatly. After the collar is put on no appearance of mutilation will be visible.

Q. How would you preserve a body that has met death by throat cutting?

A. In these cases care should be taken to tie the carotid arteries. If these vessels and the internal jugular veins have been severed, they should be secured at once. Make an incision about two and one-half inches long, severing the muscles from their attachments, and raising the integument; the common carotid artery and the internal jugular vein which is located outside it will be exposed. Tie these, and carefully inject a small quantity of fluid into the head through the carotid arteries. Inject the body through one of the same vessels. Place hardening compound in the wound to prevent putrefaction of the mutilated parts and close the cut neatly.

Q. If the heart has been taken out and the arteries which were cut tied, could a circulation through the body be obtained by use of the brachial artery?

A. Yes, a circulation might be obtained by tieing the ascending aorta and pulmonary arteries, provided those vessels had been severed near the heart, but as the ascending and descending vena cava together with the pulmonary veins have necessarily been severed in removing the heart unless these were also tied there would be so much leakage as to make it impossible to obtain a perfect circulation.

Q. If the arm were severed, one or two inches below the bend of the elbow, what arteries would be injured?

A. The radial and ulnar arteries.

Q. What arteries would you inject to determine their presence in the forearm.

A. The radial and the ulnar, raising them in the wrist.

Q. How would you secure them from leakage?

A. By a ligature. If this did not suffice, I would place a strong cord around the injured part and using a stick as a lever, twist it so tightly that no fluid could escape.

Q. If the leg were severed five or six inches below the knee, what arteries would be injured and what vessels would you inject to determine their presence?

A. The anterior and posterior tibial arteries would be injured; I would inject the femoral.

Q. When found how would you secure these arteries from leakage?

A. I should proceed as in the case of the severed arm.

Q. When both parts had been injected how would you unite them?

A. By splints and bandages, placing hardening compound between the parts to preserve the mutilated flesh.

Q. If one of the arms were severed near the trunk how would you proceed to embalm the body?

A. Tie the axillary artery and inject the body, then raise the brachial and inject the severed arm toward the distal end. When this has been done join the parts, placing hardening compound between, and neatly sew and bandage them.

Q. If called upon to care for a body where the skull was crushed and brain protruding, how would you proceed?

A. Cut across the scalp and remove it from the injured skull, raise the broken bone and remove or replace the protruding tissue of the brain. Then inject the body; if the fluid escapes remove a portion of the brain and replace it with a mixture of plaster of Paris pressed into the interior of the skull. When hardened this will prevent all leakage and the body can be embalmed. The bones of the skull should now be replaced and the scalp neatly sewed.

Q. When part of a body is mutilated what can be done to prevent putrefaction of the mutilated tissue?

A. Apply hardening compound, or a strong fluid, and bandage with surgeon's plaster; if this is not at hand, use cotton or linen bandages.

Q. If the skull has been removed for a post mortem examination, how can it be replaced without showing a mark or line across the forehead?

A. Replace the skull and fasten it with strips of surgeon's plaster, or fill the interior with putty, and place the severed portions on this. The putty will soon harden and hold the skull firmly in place.

Q. Are there any mutilated cases that cannot be embalmed arterially?

A. Yes, bodies have been so badly crushed that the bones have cut the arteries in so many places as to make it wholly impossible to obtain even a partial circulation.

Autopsy

Q. In a case of a complete autopsy when all of the organs, including the brain, have been removed from the cavities, and must be returned, how would you proceed to embalm the body and preserve the viscera?

A First, soak the viscera in a strong fluid, or, what is better, pack them in hardening compound and let them remain until the arterial embalming has been done. If the internal carotid and vertebral arteries can be found, tie them. When this is impossible, as happens frequently, mix plaster of Paris and place it in the interior of the skull pressing it down into the foramen magnum and carotid canal, through which the arteries enter the brain; when the plaster hardens it will completely close the vessels and prevent leakage. Then secure and inject the innominate artery, and the right arm, the right side of the face and a part of the right side of the body will be injected. Now inject the left carotid and the other side of the face will be preserved. The left subclavian must then be secured and injected, which will preserve the left arm and a part of that side of the body. Then raise the abdominal aorta at a point above its bifurcation, and place a large tube in it, tie the internal iliac arteries and inject toward the distal end. This operation will preserve the lower limbs and, when this is accomplished, all is done that can be done in the way of arterial embalming.

Now sponge the cavity dry, and return the abdominal and thoracic viscera to their proper places, put the brain in with them, as that organ cannot well be returned to the cranial cavity. If fluid is to be used for preserving the viscera it should be made double the usual strength. With concentrated fluid this is easy. Use fourteen ounces of chemicals instead of seven to two quarts of water. If prepared fluid is used, strengthen it with formaldehyde and chloride of zinc by adding a few ounces of each to each one-half gallon of fluid. Use a sufficient quantity of fluid to cover the viscera, and place over all a couple of layers of absorbent cotton to prevent leakage, and then after saturating the severed part sew up the body, using a fine stitch. When the skull is replaced it must be fastened as directed elsewhere, and the scalp neatly sewed together. If hardening compound is used pack the viscera in this and cover with dry saw dust. When the saw dust cannot be obtained, it may be dispensed with, and the body may be 'treated in the same manner as when fluid is used.

Signs and Tests of Death

Q. What is meant by the term apparent death?

A. That state or condition in which, while life still remains, all manifestations of it appear to be absent, and the person to all outward appearance has ceased to exist.

Q. What are the causes that lead to this condition?

A. Wagner gives the following as the principal causes: "Apparent death in consequence of internal morbid states; deep syncope, after extreme fatigue; severe spasmodic, hysterical, epileptic and eclamptic seizures; catalepsy and lethargy; many forms of yellow fever, typhoid fever and tetanus; convulsions in children; prolonged paroxysm or nervous asthma; a high degree of concussion of the brain, especially after powder explosions; wounds accompanied by much loss of blood; puerperal fever, lightning strokes and narcotic intoxication."

Q. Name all the signs of death with which you are acquainted.

Q. Cessation of heart sounds, cessation of respiration, dilatation of the pupils of the eye, a temperature much above or below normal, extreme rigidity, post mortem staining and putrefactive changes, marked by the generation of gases, discolorations, and foul odors.

Q. Give some of the tests used to ascertain if death is real or simulated.

A. Hold a light in front of the eye, and if the pupil fails to contract it is an indication that death has taken place. Hold a polished mirror over the mouth and nostrils, and observe if any moisture gathers on its surface, to indicate respiration. Place a glass of water on the chest, or better, on that portion of the body just below the breast bone, the glass being filled. If the water is spilled, it is a sign of life indicated by slight breathing.

Q. What condition of the body may be most readily mistaken for death?

A. Apoplexy, syncope, trance and asphyxia.

Q. How would you determine if a rigid state of the body was due to rigor mortis, or the rigidity of trance?

A. Break up the rigor by flexing the joints, and if it fails to return, it is rigor mortis.

Q. Give some of the more reliable tests to ascertain if the body is really dead.

A. Tie a string around the forearm or wrist sufficiently tight to prevent the blood from passing downward through the arteries. Should the parts become red or swollen above the ligature it would be an excellent sign that there was still circulation going on in the body, the swelling and color being caused by the accumulation of blood in the vessels, forced there from the arteries which are wholly or partly closed by the ligature. If no swelling or signs of redness appear the supposition is that there is no circulation, which, of course, means that death has actually taken place.

Hold a lighted candle, or fire in any form, to a part of the body and observe the effect. Should blisters form it would be a very good sign that life was not extinct. Another simple method is to rub a certain part of the body with a stiff brush or dry cloth until the epidermis comes off, and if the parts do not become moist, but on the contrary in a few hours become dry and hard, it is an indication that death has taken place. A mustard plaster is sometimes applied to the skin of the body as a simple test. In cases of real death the spot where the mustard lay does not become red, as it always does in life.

Post mortem discolorations caused by blood in the superficial veins, from which the oxygen has escaped, carrying the hemoglobin or coloring matter of the blood with it, and staining the parts over the course of the vessel, is a good sign that death has actually taken place.

Q. Are there any positive signs of death.

A. Yes, one. The visible presence of putrefaction, marked by the accumulation of gases, chemical discolorations and foul odors.

Q. If after making tests the embalmer is still in doubt as to the actual presence of death what course should he pursue?

A. Immediately notify the attending physician, who should be much better qualified to judge than himself. Let him decide and take the responsibility.

Section IV - The Funeral Director

Q. What qualities should an up-to-date funeral director possess?

A. The Rev. Stephen Merritt, one of the Nestors of the funeral directors of the city of New York, says that like an artist or a poet, an undertaker is born, not made, and I think this is true. A man, however rough or uncouth, may perform the functions of a funeral director, but unless he is born with the necessary natural abilities, though he may do his best to fit himself for a position which nature never intended him to fill, he will never be more than mediocre in his profession. Every undertaker should be a gentleman both by nature and by cultivation, but if he lacks the attributes of a gentleman he should at least try to assume the appearance of one while conducting his business. He should have full command of himself at all times and in all places, never bluster, brag, or use profane or obscene language. In person, a funeral director, like any other professional man, should be scrupulously clean, and well but not flashily dressed. I am frequently asked if an undertaker should always wear a Prince Albert coat and a silk hat. I should reply that in my judgment this depends very much upon the man and the locality. While conducting a funeral a man to whom such a coat is becoming, and who becomes the coat, should certainly wear it, and if a silk hat is likewise becoming, wear that. Every man engaged in the business should be a rule unto himself as regards his personal appearance. It is sufficient if he is neatly and becomingly dressed in a manner suited to himself and to his calling. A funeral director need not be a scholar, at least so far as book learning is concerned, but all men of education are not necessarily graduates of universities. A man with a common school education and a goodly fund of general knowledge may consistently be called an educated man. However, the funeral director's education is not complete without a general knowledge of anatomy, physiology and sanitary science. A successful undertaker must be a good business man; like all men of business, he should be able to figure profit and loss, and consider the profit he must make on his average funeral to pay a fair return on the capital invested, to pay for his personal services and those of his assistant or assistants, and to compensate for the deterioration in his rolling stock, horses and other paraphernalia, the last being one of the largest items of expense of the modern funeral director and very often overlooked when figuring his annual profits. Many undertakers lay the cause of their failure to succeed to excessive competition and are constantly asking for -laws designed to prohibit, or at least deter others from entering the business, forgetting the law of the survival of the fittest, and that the best and only way to deal with competition is to make one's services so valuable, and one's self personally so agreeable to the public that the newcomer will soon learn that the people have no use for his services and will quit the field. The writer is personally acquainted with an undertaker who has the whole business of a small city because his services are so acceptable to the public that whenever competition has been contemplated, would-be competitors have been warned by some citizen that it would be impossible for them to gain a foothold so great is the popularity of the present incumbent.

Q. How should the office of a modern funeral director be arranged?

A. In most undertaking establishments the office and reception room are necessarily the same, and for that reason the office should be made as attractive as possible without being showy. The office furniture should be of good, but not necessarily of costly material. Flowers in an office make it look attractive, but there should not be too large a quantity of these, and in a small office palms look out of place. A sufficient number of chairs should always be in the office for the accommodation of visitors who call on business, and pretty but not gaudy pictures may be placed on the walls. A good roll-top desk and a small library may complete the office fixtures.

Q. Are cabinets for holding caskets desirable?

A. That like many other arrangements is a matter of individual taste and convenience. If the funeral director has plenty of room it is much better to display his caskets on pedestals, or what is better, light table-like frames, which can be placed on little trucks, making it easier to move the casket at convenience, from one part of the room to another. The room where the display is made should be as nearly dustproof as possible and covers should be provided for each casket. This makes the most attractive show-room and, with the different qualities of goods set out before them, gives the purchaser a chance to compare styles and prices. At the present time many caskets are bought already trimmed, and when set out in this way make as attractive an appearance as it is possible to make of such goods as coffins and caskets.

Q. Suppose you had an undertaking and furniture business would you advertise the two kinds of business together?

A. As before stated, an up-to-date professional man never advertises his business. When a physician resorts to advertising he is rated as a quack, no matter if he be a graduate of a reputable medical school. It is perfectly proper for an undertaker and furniture dealer to use a card as such, but he should never advertise his prices, facilities or professional services. Let your abilities speak for themselves; if you are the right man in the right place the public will soon learn of it and appreciate you accordingly. A furniture dealer may and generally finds it necessary to advertise whether he is a funeral director or not.

Q. The new transportation rules forbid the shipping of the remains of persons dead of certain diseases. Name those diseases.

A. The new shipping rules prohibit only smallpox and bubonic plague. The old rules prohibited smallpox, Asiatic cholera, yellow and typhus fever and bubonic plague. These rules were revised in 1903 and the new rules were approved by the American Association of Baggage Agents, the Conference of State and Provincial Boards of Health, and the National Funeral Directors' Association, and are now in force in many of the States.

Q. What kind of crepe should be hung on the door when death has entered a home?

A. This is a matter of taste and custom which varies with different communities and should be left largely to the friends of the deceased. In most places the custom is to use white for persons under twenty years of age, and a mixture of black and white for persons whose ages vary between twenty and iqrty years. For persons above forty years of age, black is most in use, but in cases of women, especially, a mixture of colors, such as black and purple for people of advanced age, and silver gray for those dying in middle life is in good taste. In many of the larger cities, wreaths of flowers are used on the door in place of crepe. In this case they may be made of either white or colored flowers with ribbon of suitable color.

Q. Should relatives of the deceased act as pall-bearers?

A. When the writer was a young man the custom of near relatives acting in the capacity of pall-bearers had never been heard of, but at the present time many families think it is the proper thing for the nearest relatives and friends to bear the bodies of their loved ones to their final resting place. Whether this be advisable or not depends upon the conditions in individual cases. In case of the death of a parent having four stalwart sons there would seem to be nothing more consistent and appropriate than that the body of the father or mother should be borne by them to its resting place. But the custom of requesting the nearest relatives to perform this duty regardless of age or physical condition is, in my judgment, out of taste, it being next to impossible to find from four to six near relatives of the deceased physically capable of performing the duty.

Q. Where the body is that of an elderly person should old men be selected as pall-bearers?

A. If it is the expressed wish of the family, and elderly but vigorous men can be found who are able and willing to perform the duty, no objections should be raised by the funeral director, but generally speaking, young men are much to be preferred; they are much better fitted for it physically, and are much quicker to comprehend what is required of them, and will invariably perform their duty in a more quiet and less obtrusive manner than older men.

Q. Should the pall-bearers be instructed by the funeral director in relation to their duties?

A. In case the business of the undertaker is such as to warrant the expense he should have paid and drilled pallbearers who are ready to respond to his call at short notice. This simplifies his duties and helps things to move on smoothly, while undrilled men are constantly getting out of place, and in each other's way, causing much annoyance to the director and disturbing the smooth and even conduct of the proceedings. Where this is not possible and untrained men must be used, as is usually the case, the funeral director should spend some time after the bearers are selected in instructing them as to their duties. If the funeral is to be conducted at the house, instruct them as to the positions they are to take, and how the casket can best be removed, how to place it in the hearse, and what carriage they are to occupy, if any. When at the church, instruct them how to carry and place the casket, and what pews they are to occupy. When church trucks are used the bearers should always precede it and be seated at once, those on the left taking the second pew and those on the right the front one.

Q. Should the pall-bearers lower the body into the grave?

A. Lowering devices have now become so common that in most cases this service is not needed. However, if they are not used, unless there are attendants in the cemetery to do this, the bearers should attend to it. When, the device is used and they have deposited the casket at the grave, they should walk back to the entrance to the cemetery and arrange themselves on either side of the gate, remaining there until the procession passes out.

Q. What is the meaning of the word undertaker?

A. Originally the word meant one who undertook to do something that nobody else wanted to do. The present meaning of the word is, of course, well known.

Q. When an undertaker is called to a case what paraphernalia is it necessary for him to take with him?

A. He should take a cooling board and an embalming cabinet, the latter containing all necessary instruments — embalming fluid, disinfectants, comb, brush, razor, bandages, sponges, absorbent cotton, soaps, towels, cosmetics, such as complexion tints and powders, and other articles too numerous to mention. A couple of rubber blankets for use in case of emergency is an indispensable part of an undertakers and embalmer's outfit, and a pair of sheets are an excellent addition, as these are articles which are often soiled while a body is being embalmed, and if they are one's own property they can be taken away, thereby saving embarrassment and preventing the danger of questions being asked by the friends which one would not care to answer. At the first call crepe should always be placed on the door, whether at request or not; this can be changed later if necessary.

Q. Is placing caskets in the show windows of an up-to-date undertaking establishment to be commended or discouraged?

A. That is a matter for each funeral director to decide for himself, but in my judgment the day for the undertaker to pose as a business man or to practise the methods of a shopkeeper has gone by, and should be avoided by all up-to-date professional men. Almost everybody can read, and the sign funeral director and embalmer may be appropriately placed over the door and upon the windows of the establishment, and no other indication of his business need be displayed. Should I pass the office of a physician, and see bottles of medicine and surgical instruments conspicuously placed in a show window I should take it for granted that the occupant of the office was a quack. The funeral director of the present day is either a business man or a professional man, and he should choose between the two. If he is a business man he has a right to call the attention of the public to his wares in any honorable and lawful way, either by a display of goods or by advertising how low his prices are and how cheap his services can be obtained. But, if he is a professional man, he should never use the methods of the shopkeeper, but let his goods and professional services speak for themselves.

Q. When the funeral is held at the house what position should the casket occupy in the room?

A. A great deal depends upon the room, and on whether it is to be a public or a private funeral. It is no longer considered improper not to place the casket in the center of the room, and space can be saved by placing it near the wall, either at the end, side or across a corner. The flowers take up much room, as they are now being made almost entirely in set pieces, and if put in the center of the room of an ordinary apartment, especially in our cities, would not leave room enough for the relatives and near friends. If placed across the corner there is space left at the back of the casket for quite a display of flowers and the effect is very good; if the minister stands at the head, that leaves almost the entire room for the immediate friends. There are the same advantages in placing the casket at the end or side of the room with the exception of not having the corner for the flowers. A small space should always be left between the casket and the wall, which is usually filled up with flowers.

Q. How should a body be placed in the casket?

A. After the embalming is done and the body is dressed and ready for the casket, to lift and lay it in the proper position would appear to be a simple task, and yet it is one that the amateur sometimes does in a very awkward manner, and if he begin awkwardly he is liable to continue in that way. Place the head of the embalming board at the foot of the casket, either parallel with it or at a right angle. Then place the right arm beneath the neck, placing the hand beneath the left shoulder blade, letting the head and neck of the body rest on the middle of the arm, and place the left arm beneath the body. Your assistant should place his left arm beneath the knees and with the right grasp the lower extremities, and in this way carry the body to, and place it in, the casket, taking care not to disturb the lining more than is necessary. The position of the body in the casket is of much importance, as it may appear to be in a cramped or awkward position. The head should never be raised too high to have the appearance of ease in sleep, or placed so low as to appear to h& uncomfortable if the position were that of one sleeping in life.

When everything is arranged to your satisfaction, request the friends to step in and view the body in the casket, and ask if they have any suggestions to make, and if so satisfy them if possible, even if their taste does not agree with your own.

Q. How can the draping of a body be best accomplished?

A. As canopies are fast becoming a thing of the past, a good idea is to be provided with three snow-white linen sheets. Cover the cooling board with one, allowing the edges to reach the floor. Place the body with the head as it will be when on the pillow in the casket. Then put a pillow under the head and another lengthwise under the legs below the knees; this will take away the prominence of the feet. Double the second sheet lengthwise; lift the body and slip the folded side under the shoulder, having the edges reach the floor at the head; cross the ends of the sheet over the breast, being careful not to draw it too tight, as the edge of the sheet must form right angles on the floor corresponding with the cooling board. Place the other sheet over the body, folding the hem under the chin and allowing the sides to reach the floor, pinning the ends to the end of sheet number two. This will give a couch-like effect and will be very pleasing.

Q. When the jaw falls, how can the mouth be successfully closed?

A. On this question there are many different opinions. Some use a chin rest until the body is embalmed, and expect that the embalming fluid will cause the jaw to set so firmly that it will remain in place, arid condemn the fluid if it does not. Others inject formaldehyde, full strength, into the mouth at the condyle of the lower jaw, causing the external pterygoid muscle to harden and set the jaw firmly in place. Experiments have proven that this will sometimes work well, but at other times will fail. When the chin rest is used, a cotton pad should be placed under the chin so that no indentation will be made by the contact of the instrument with the skin. The best way to hold a jaw in place is with a stitch made in the following manner: Using a half-curve needle and a strong thread, pass it under the ligament in the center of the lower jaw, beneath the under lip, then upwards beneath the upper lip to one of the nostrils, then draw the thread through and pass the needle through the septum, separating the two nostrils, keeping the needle close to the jaw, now pass it downwards beneath the upper lip, and after raising the jaw to its natural position, hold it there, and tie the thread; in this way the jaw will always remain in place, and if the work is properly done, there will be no puckering or drawing of the lip or other unnatural expression of the mouth. The only objection that can be urged against this method is the fact that some lips naturally part in life, and of course will and should do so after death, thus showing the thread. In this case, a wire staple can be used which inserted in the upper and lower jaw will lock them together. When this device is used always place the fastening under the cheeks. When the lips naturally part, as indicated above, the best way is to leave them so, but some people will insist upon having them closed and their wishes must, of course, be gratified. This can usually be accomplished by using the stitch without passing the needle through the septum of the nose, but by passing it under the ligament in the center of the upper jaw, under the lip. This will draw the lips together and usually close them, but a drawn appearance of the mouth cannot be avoided, and it will look much better if left as nature made it.

Q. How should the eyes be closed?

A. First wash the eyeball and inside of the lid with fluid. This can be done with the forceps using a small piece of cotton. Then wipe it dry with a piece of soft muslin or absorbent cotton, held in the forceps, raise the lower lid and draw down the upper one to meet it. The eyes will then remain closed. Never lap the upper over the lower lid, as it gives an unnatural appearance. If the eyeball is sunken, raise the lid with pads of absorbent cotton or eye-caps. This, if skillfully done, will give the desired fullness and hold the lids closed. Never resort to injecting the eyeball as advocated by some, for it is a dangerous practice. I once had occasion to fix a body which had been embalmed and shipped from Germany to New York. The body had been dead three months, but was in a state of perfect preservation except that the eyes had wholly disappeared. I filled the sockets with soft putty, moulded to about the natural size of the eye, then drew up the lower lid carefully, and the upper one down to meet it, and held them in position until the putty hardened; this kept them closed and gave a perfectly natural appearance to the eyes.

Q. What are the first duties of a funeral director on the day when he is to conduct a funeral at the home of the deceased?

A. Let us suppose that the time for the funeral is set for two o'clock in the afternoon. The funeral director should be at the house as early as ten o'clock. He should consult with the friends and make all necessary arrangements in regard to placing the casket, locating the clergyman and singers, also placing chairs, arranging flowers and looking after such other details as seem to be necessary, such as arranging the carriage list, planning his way out with the casket, and instructing the pall-bearers in their duties. Early attention to these details make it easy to conduct a funeral smoothly and leaves a lasting impression on the minds of the relatives and friends as to the executive ability of the undertaker.

Q. What are the duties of the funeral director on arriving at the house in the afternoon.

A. To verify his carriage list and to take a general survey of everything and see that all is in order. He should then stand at the door prepared to receive the friends. If the weather is cold he should attend to the door, opening and closing it as gently and quietly as possible. While he is receiving guests at the door, it is well to have a lady or gentleman assistant to conduct them to their seats. On the arrival of the clergyman and singers he should conduct them to their respective places and when all is in readiness, quietly notify the clergyman that he may proceed. After which he should resume his place at the door to admit late comers.

Q. After the service what is the next duty of the undertaker?

A. Provided services are not to be held at the grave, to conduct the minister and singers to the carriages provided for their use, and to instruct the driver to drive them to their homes, and if the carriages are to be made further use of, to return as quickly as possible. He should then return to the house and announce to the friends that an opportunity will now be given them to view the remains. This notice should be given to one apartment at a time in order to avoid confusion.

Q. In what order should the carriages be announced?

A. That depends upon the taste of the funeral director. Many prefer to announce the carriage of the nearest relatives first, while other excellent and popular undertakers call the carriage that is to be last in the procession first, and after seeing the relatives seated therein order it moved on two carriage lengths and then allow each successive carriage to pass on and take its position in front of the former one until the procession is formed. This they say allows the immediate relatives a few moments alone with their dead, which is very pleasing to them. After the carriages are formed in line the casket should be placed in the hearse, the director immediately superintending the removal of it, after which he may remove the crepe from the door, place pedestals and rugs out of view and return to his carriage, which should always be placed at the head of the procession, the pall-bearers immediately following in front of the hearse.

Q. How should the grave be prepared for the reception of the body?

A. The walls of the grave should be lined with bleached sheeting, which can be fastened with wire nails driven into the soil, or trimmed with evergreen, which is much to be preferred in country towns in the East where evergreen trees abound. A modern lowering device should always be used, and should be neatly covered. The earth removed by digging the grave should be hidden by a grass-green cloth or evergreen bows, as all these things tend to lessen the horror of the grave and assuage the grief of those who mourn. Arriving at the grave the casket should be removed from the hearse and placed on the lowering device. The flowers should be spread on the covering of the mound. Then the hearse should move forward and the director should ask the relatives if they wish to alight, and if so, assist them to do so. If they do not wish to, the pall-bearers should arrange themselves on either side of the drive near to the gate and the procession be allowed to pass through.

Q. How should a church funeral be conducted?

A. (Answered by J. Frank Childs.) "Previous to the time of the funeral I have ordered all flowers, except those destined to remain on the casket, to be taken to the church, where I repair with my church truck, for which I have a black and a white drape. After placing it in the most convenient place in the vestibule to receive the casket, I arrange the flowers around the platform as best I can. I have ascertained how many seats will be occupied by the mourners, and draw a white ribbon to designate them. I usually reserve the front seats on the right of the middle aisle for them, and opposite seats for organizations. Arriving at the church the hearse is drawn to one side and I immediately assist the mourners out of the hacks, instructing them to form in procession in the vestibule and await my coming. When all have been assisted out I repair to the right of the procession and conduct them slowly to their seats, removing the ribbon as I pass down and seating them as nearly as possible as they were seated in the carriages. I then retire, remove the casket from the hearse and place it on the bier, arranging the flowers on the casket. If organizations are in attendance, they now file into their seats and remain standing until the casket is in position. The bearers precede the casket down the aisle and open ranks, allowing me to pass through. I place the casket, remove the lid, the bearers file to their seats and I give a nod to the minister to proceed with the service. At its close I arrange everything about the casket and announce in a quiet way that those present desiring to take leave of their friend will now have the opportunity. Passing down one outside aisle and out by way of the other, I lead them to the casket, the procession always passing from foot to head, and take my position near the mourners, remaining standing until ail have passed out, the organizations being the last in the procession. I then announce to the mourners that they will take leave of their friend and resume their seats, always giving them ample time. I return, have the carriages drawn up, reconduct the mourners out, assist them into their respective carriages and then proceed to the cemetery."

Q. What position in the funeral procession should the honorary pallbearers occupy?

A. Behind the minister and preceding the active pallbearers.

Q. Is it proper for the director to order the hearse to be backed up to the curb to receive the casket, or should it be left standing in or beside the street?

A. Most funeral directors think that the hearse should stand at the side of the street nearest the house or church, but in some places the hearse is backed up to the curb, and on the whole I think that custom the most sensible, as it certainly saves the bearers a lift of several inches, besides saving them the necessity of stepping into the street when the streets are in bad condition.

Q. Where is the proper place for the funeral director in the church?

A. At the rear of the church where he can observe the proceedings.

Q. Should a body be dressed immediately after embalming?

A. It is not advisable. No one can tell what trouble may ensue later.

Q. If called to attend a funeral in the country as the director only, and on arrival at the house you found the body purging, what would you do?

A. First ascertain the cause, which is probably gas in the stomach or lungs. If so, relieve it. You should always carry an emergency case of instruments for this purpose. If you have none, a pocket knife can be used in the stomach to relieve the gas. When the trouble is in the lungs pressure can be used on the chest, causing the mucous to escape from the mouth and nostrils, which can be taken up with a sponge, and may relieve the trouble temporarily. But the best way is always to have your operating case with you.

Q. How would you keep false teeth in the mouth of a dead body?

A. Wipe the mouth as dry as possible with a soft muslin or cotton, cover the plate with Le Page's glue, or some other good cement, place the teeth in position and hold them there until the cement hardens.

Q. What is the best position for flowers at a funeral?

A. In most cases the family, or someone in charge, will wish to decide, otherwise use your own judgment. The flowers placed on the casket had best be left there if possible until it is lowered into the grave; if there are more than can be carried on the casket they can be placed in the carriage designed for the pall bearers, if there is not a special carriage for them. After the burial the flowers should be placed on and around the grave.

Q. At a house funeral when should the friends be allowed to view the remains?

A. Different customs prevail in different localities. Some funeral directors require the friends to view the remains on entering the house, the family having previously taken their leave, after which the casket is closed and not reopened; 'others keep the casket closed to the end of the service and then offer the friends an opportunity to view the remains, after which the family take their leave. If no regular custom prevails, the best way is to consult the wishes of the relatives.

Q. What soil is the most favorable for cemeteries?

A. Probably sandy soil, as the grave will be less likely to contain water, and is more easily dug; and it is said that sandy or gravelly soil acts as a filterer for impurities; however, if the cemetery is far removed from streams, as it always should be, this will make but little difference.

Q. How soon should you bury a body after death caused by a contagious disease?

A. As soon as convenient for the family, but if necessary to keep it, and permission is granted, I would not hesitate to say that I could make it innocuous to the living for any reasonable period of time.

Q. In the absence of external wounds how would you determine whether death was the result of violent or natural causes?

A. If impossible to judge from circumstances, the only way is through a post mortem examination.

Q. Do you think it wise to allow the friends to remain in the room while preparing the body?

A. Generally speaking, it is much better to educate the friends to allow the undertaker and his assistants the room to themselves while embalming or dressing a body, but it is hard to make an iron rule; to positively forbid them entrance arouses suspicion and may create hard feelings. If a relative or friend insists upon being present, he or she should be allowed to do so, but be careful what you do in their presence.

Q. What bodies may be shipped under Rule 2.

A. See transportation rules.

Q. Is it possible to tell a good from a poor fluid without experimenting with it?

A. Not without having it analyzed, and even then one would want to know the effects of certain chemicals on dead tissue, and be well informed as to the germicidal powers of the antiseptics it contained.

Q. *a* What class of embalmers can ship under Rule 2? *b* Remains dead of what disease are shipped under Rule 2? *c* In what do the requirements for a licensed and a non-licensed embalmer differ under Rule 3? *d* What are the requirements of Rule 8? *e* What advantage has the licensed over the unlicensed embalmer under Rule 8?

A. 'See transportation rules.

Q. Is an undertaker liable to prosecution for shipping a body dead of a contagious disease when the physician reports it not contagious or infectious?

A. No; he has only to show the death certificate; the responsibility rests with the physician.

Q. Is it necessary to disinfect the hearse and other carriages used where death is caused by a contagious disease? If so, under what circumstances should it be done and how would you do it?

A. If the body had been placed in the casket without having first been disinfected, or if the casket had been exposed to the germs of the disease before the room was disinfected, then it would be necessary to disinfect the hearse; otherwise it would not. If the friends and their clothing had been exposed in the sick room, or other infected apartments it would be necessary to disinfect carriages in which they had driven, otherwise it would be unnecessary. A closed hearse or closed carriages may be disinfected by the use of a small formaldehyde lamp. If the carriages are open, place them in as close an apartment as possible, and after disinfecting leave them out of doors in the open air and sunshine.

Q. What bodies are forbidden shipment by the rules of many of the State Boards of Health?

A. Bodies dead of smallpox, Asiatic cholera, bubonic plague and typhus fever.

Q. What precautions would you take in disinterring a body dead of smallpox?

A. The probabilities are that the Board of Health would not permit such a body to be exhumed, especially if it could not be shown that the body had been thoroughly disinfected before burial, but if it were permitted, extra precaution should be used. The person doing the work should be an immune if possible, and should wear an old suit of clothes, as they should be immediately destroyed. A large quantity of a solution of bichloride of mercury, 1:500, should be used to sprinkle the soil near the receptacle containing the body, after which the casket, box or coffin, and afterwards the remains, should be thoroughly disinfected, by sprinkling with the same disinfectant. The body should then be removed in a metal-lined receptacle. After the work is done, all clothing or fabrics used or worn should be destroyed by fire, and the body or bodies of those participating in the work should be thoroughly disinfected.

Q. What qualities should a good embalming fluid possess?

A. It should be a good preservative, disinfectant and deodorizer, and the chemicals of which it is composed should be of such a nature as to give the best possible appearance to the face or other exposed parts of the body.

Q. What is the objection to arsenic in embalming fluids?

A. Its use may defeat the ends of justice, or cast unjust suspicion in cases where arsenical poisoning is suspected.

Q. What would you do to prevent dessication of the lips after embalming?

A. The application of a little vaseline or the use of a wet cloth will prevent dessication of the lips, or any other part of the body.

Q. Would the means used interfere with the proper appearance of the body?

A. Certainly not; the vaseline may be easily removed by a sponge wet with alcohol.

Q. What is decomposition and how is it detected?

A. Nature's chemical process of returning a dead body to its original elements; putrefaction, accompanied by fermentation, caused by the putrefactive bacteria under the influence of heat and moisture, detected by the presence of gas, discolorations, and bad odors.

Q. In what bodies does putrefaction progress most rapidly?

A. In bodies dead of blood poisoning in any form; puerperal fever, alcoholism, erysipelas, uremic poisoning, typhoid fever, and peritonitis; drowned and dropsical cases are often classed among bodies that decompose rapidly, but they are easily preserved after the water has been removed.

Q. What is an immune?

A. A person not liable to take a contagious disease by reason of having previously been afflicted with it, by reason of acclimation or by vaccination.

Q. Is there any other way by which a body can be thoroughly embalmed, except by arterial injection?

A. A body may be preserved for an indefinite period of time by needle, cavity and hypodermic work, but a body so treated is not thoroughly or safely embalmed.

Q. What is meant by dessication?

A. Drying up of the tissues.

Q. How soon after death should a body be embalmed?

A. As early as convenient after the body has been placed on an incline and the blood allowed to drain from the exposed parts. Provided, always, that there is no doubt about the actual presence of death.

Q. If a body is taken from the water, how would you determine whether death was caused from drowning or from some other cause?

A. Water in the air cells of the lungs is an indication that drowning is the cause of death, but should the water be absent it is by no means certain that life was extinct before the body entered the water. If there were external indications of violence, the absence of water in the lungs would be strong corroborative evidence that the cause of death was not drowning.

Q. What restrictions are imposed by most of the Boards of Health on shipping bodies dead of a contagious disease?

A. Smallpox and bubonic plague are forbidden shipment, and most of the boards refuse to allow the shipment of any body dead of a contagious disease, unless it is prepared by a licensed embalmer.

Q. What causes discolorations?

A. Usually blood in the superficial vessels, but it may be the result of disease, such as jaundice, Addison's disease, or the spots of purpura; they are also sometimes the results of chemical changes, which cannot be satisfactorily accounted for.

Q. What steps should be taken to secure transportation of a disinterred body?

A. Comply with the rules of the local Board of Health, with which every undertaker should be familiar.

Q. How long does it take for the soft parts of a body to decompose?

A. That depends on the condition of the body, the kind of soil in which buried, and upon whether or not it has been embalmed. No one can tell how long the soft or other parts may last after burial. I once saw a body raised fourteen days after burial and seventeen days after death, which had not been embalmed, and it was in a perfect state of preservation. This was probably due to the chemical condition of the body, and the soil in which it was buried. The body was that of an old and fleshy lady whose weight was about one hundred and eighty pounds.

Q. What is the cause of the phenomenon known as skin-slipping, or more properly slipping of the epidermis?

A. Slipping of the epidermis is caused first by putrefaction of the fatty tissues beneath the skin, which spreads to and involves the epidermis, and affects the rete mucosum, softening that substance and causing the cuticle to slip from its attachment to the true skin.

Q. What disinterred bodies are dangerous to the public health?

A. All, especially those dead of a contagious disease, and those buried but a few months.

Q. What are the duties of a shipping undertaker when death has been caused by scarlet fever?

A. To see that the body is properly embalmed and disinfected, and all of the rules of the Board of Health complied with; to notify the receiving undertaker by mail of the time of shipment and when the body may be expected to arrive; acquaint him with what has been done, the kind of fluid and disinfectants used, etc.

Q. What would be the duty of the receiving undertaker in such a case?

A. To notify the health authorities of the receipt of the case, and all the facts connected therewith, and, if it were the desire of the friends to view the remains, to apply for permission to allow them to do so; to notify the shipping undertaker of the receipt and condition of the body, and of any other facts that may be of interest or profit to him.

Q. Has the attending physician the right to hold an autopsy on a body without consulting the funeral director in charge?

A. The funeral director would have no authority in the matter, but it would be wisdom on the part of the undertaker to try and persuade the physician to allow him to embalm the body before the post mortem was performed, as it would save a great deal of trouble.

Q. I wish to ship a body that has been in a vault ten days. I employ you as my undertaker. Describe minutely what you would do.

A. First, ascertain the cause of death and then apply to the Board of Health for a permit to remove the remains. When this is obtained, treat the body as a contagious case, observing all the rules of the Board of Health in your city or town, and also those of the State or locality to which the body is to be shipped.

Q. Would you take care of a body dead of smallpox?

A. Not if it could possibly be avoided. There is usually an immune in the town and he should be employed to look after a body dead of this disease, under the direction of the Board of Health. It is probable that no embalming would be allowed and consequently no skill required.

Women as Embalmers

Q. Should lady embalmers and lady assistants be encouraged by the profession?

A. Having been asked to answer the above question, I herewith reply, speaking from my seven years' experience as a lady embalmer.

When death enters the home, and robs it of mother, daughter or prattling babe, the bereaved family naturally turn to a sympathetic friend for advice and assistance.

At that time a lady embalmer may not only perform her necessary duties for the departed one, but by her tender and solicitous care for the comfort and assistance of those who mourn, she will prove a blessing and surely a friend never to be forgotten.

Are our loved ones not as sacred in death as in life, and should we allow the opposite sex to perform work at that time, which we would not allow in life?

The question, "If a nurse washes and prepares a body for the undertaker, why is a lady embalmer required?" is often asked. Every member of the profession certainly knows, or should know, that a gentleman called upon to do

145

the embalming may just as well do all the work as part of it; there is no dividing line; a lady embalmer should perform the entire work from the time she is called in until the body is placed in the casket.

When an experienced woman is in charge, the family, having full confidence in her ability, give the care of their dear ones to her, knowing she will arrange the clothes, dress the hair and attend to the minor details as she would for her own.

Should the lady embalmer be encouraged by the profession? Yes, a lady who not only understands the art and science of embalming, but who is expert in all the other details of the work, by her kind and sympathetic manner to the bereaved can comfort them in their sorrow and is by all means a necessity and a growing need.

Has the business reached the high goal entitling it to be called a profession? At the present day, decidedly no; had it attained that elevated standard, lady embalmers would btr constantly sought for, but at the present time, the undertakers are jealously guarding every entrance by which a woman may enter this path of duty.

When the lady embalmer is recognized by the undertaker it will be an evidence that it is worthy to be called a profession; for the gentle and refining influence of successful ladies in the business, will raise the public estimate and tend to elevate the business to a profession in its true sense, and make it an art which any true participant should be proud to practice, and a profession in which any lady would certainly not be ashamed to be engaged.

Mrs. Harry Mason White.

Dressing a Body

Q. Explain in detail how you would proceed to dress and prepare a body for the casket, stating the proper time, place, etc.

A. The best time for dressing a body seems, for many reasons, to be that of laying out, and the best place the room in which it is to remain. Moving the body after it has been dressed is liable to much inconvenience, as the clothes become displaced and the hair disarranged. Several advantages are gained by dressing a body soon after death; it is more pliable at this time; skin-slipping, which may take place two or three days after death, will not then have occurred, and, more important still, it is likely to give better satisfaction to relatives and friends, those most intimately concerned. They will wish to see it early, and where the body has been already dressed, the effect will be less startling. In some cases, of course, where the clothes are not in readiness or the family actually desire delay, one must yield to necessity; in this case, the body should be dressed just before it is to be laid in the casket.

One should endeavor to have the apartment to one's self while dressing the body. The presence of others in the room is open to the same objections as while embalming the body. The body should be placed on a level, with the head resting on a pillow. The first thing to be done is to remove the rigor mortis by flexing fingers and joints, working the arms gently outward and upward. Sometimes, too, the stiffness of the neck may be removed in the same way.

Where a winding sheet is used, it should be arranged by one who has some skill in drapery. With a sheet of soft material, beautiful effects can be produced by an artistic hand. The goods should be gathered into the hand halfway down the sheet, and the folds laid beneath the neck. The sheet should then be drawn down beneath the body to the thighs, and the ends brought down over the shoulders to the feet. The goods can be draped about the arms and pinned in such a way as to give the graceful flowing effect of the sleeves of college gowns. The size of the sheet, of course, must depend upon the size of the person; for one of medium stature it should be from two to three yards in length and two yards wide. The winding sheet, though less in use than formerly, is an excellent substitute for the robe, which seldom fits, and often does not fasten in the back.

Women are usually laid out in night robes, which are left on the body when it is dressed. A convenient way to put on the waist is to lay it upside down and slip the arms in first; then raise the arms over the head, and lifting the body or rolling it gently from side to side slip the waist under the shoulders. Skirts should be put on, one inside the other, and slipped up, all at once, over the limbs. The arrangement of the hair is of great importance in dressing the bodies of women. It should be done in the same way as worn in life. It should be arranged when the body has been dressed, preferably, by a friend; otherwise the undertaker or his representative, a woman, if possible, should make sure he understands the way the subject customarily wore it.

The bodies of men are dressed in much the same way as those of women. The under and outer shirts may often be put one inside the other, and be put on at the same time. They can be best put on in the same way as the woman's waist is adjusted. Hold the shirt upside down, the neck toward the feet, and draw the arms through the sleeves. Slip the shirt down over the head. It is often best before putting on the shirt to place a towel over the face and draw it in under the chin. This will prevent the shirt from injuring the face as it is slipped on. The drawers and trousers may be drawn up over the limbs by lifting the body slightly. The collar and tie should be put on next; the vest and coat may be adjusted in the same way as the shirt. Avoid cutting the garments, if possible, and when absolutely necessary, be sure to secure the cuts by sewing or pinning with safety pins.

The essentials in successful dressing are a deft hand, some practice, good taste and good sense.. Details of procedure will differ with individual cases, but these general methods, if pursued, will be found helpful.

A FRIEND.

Dictionary of Anatomical Words and Phrases

Ab-dō'mĕn. The cavity bounded above by the diaphragm and below by the pelvis.

Ab-dŏm'ĭ-nal. Pertaining to the abdomen.

Ab-dŭc'tor. A muscle which serves to draw a part outward.

Ab-nor'mal. Not according to rule; irregular.

A-brās'ion. A removal of the cuticle in any manner, as by rubbing.

Abs'cĕss. An inflammatory or purulent tumor; a gathering, or bou.

Ab-sorb'. To suck up, as with a sponge.

Ab-sorb'ents. Vessels or glands which absorb. Dressings which absorb liquids or gases.

Ab-sorp'tion. Act of absorbing.

Ac-cum'ul-ate. To collect; to gather.

A-cĕt'ic. Relating to vinegar or having similar properties.

A-cĕt'ic Acid. The acid which is the chief ingredient in vinegar.

Ac-ro'mĭ-ŏn. The upper process of the shoulder-blade artictdating with the collar-bone.

A-cūte'. Quick; sharp; as a quick, sharp pain. Opposed to chronic; as an acute disease.

Ad-dūce'. To bring forward; to advance; to urge.

Ad-dŭc'tor. A muscle that draws forward, or brings parts of the body together.

Ad-dŭc'tor Lon'gus. Muscle on inside of thigh.

Ad-hēre'. To stick to, as wax to the finger; to be closely united.

Ad-hē'sion. The act or state of adhering.

A-dŭl'ter-āte. To corrupt by some foreign mixture.

A-e-ro'bic. Pertaining to microbes which are dependent upon oxygen for life.

Af-fect'ed. Acted upon; having produced an effect or change.

A'gue. An intermittent fever, in which cold fits alternate with hot.

Air Cell. A receptacle for air in various parts of the system, as a cavity in the cellular tissue of the lungs.

Al-bū'men / Al-bū'min. The white of an egg. A constituent of all animal bodies.

Al-bū'min-ate. Compound of albumen and certain bases, as albuminate of iron.

Al'ka-lĭ. A basic compound which neutralizes acids, unites with fats to form soap, and turns reddened litmus blue.

Al'ka-līne. Having the properties of an alkali.

Al-lŏ-trŏp'ic. Pertaining to allotropism.

Al-lŏt'rŏp-ism. The existence in nature of the same substance in two or more different forms of varying physical properties.

Al-vě'ō-lar. Relating to the sockets of the teeth.

Am-mō'nǐ-a (NH3). A gaseous substance formed by the union of nitrogen and hydrogen.

Am'ni-ŏn. The membrane that surrounds the foetus in the womb.

Am'ni-ŏt'ic. Of, or pertaining to the amnion; as the amniotic fluid.

A-nae'mi-a. A morbid condition in which the blood is deficient in quantity or quality.

An-aes-thět'ǐc. A substance used to produce insensibility to pain.

An'a-lyze. To resolve a compound into its elementary parts.

A-nŏm'a-ly. Unusual condition.

An-a-sar'ca. General dropsy.

A-năs'tō-mōse. To unite, as vessels or branches, with one another.

An-as'to-mŏt'i-ca Mag'na. One of the branches of the brachial artery.

A-năt'o-my. The science of the structure of organized bodies.

An-ti-sěp'tic. A drug or chemical which checks or retards putrefaction.

An'thrăx. Carbuncle; a painful, dark-colored tumor.

An'eū-rism. A soft tumor, containing blood, caused by the rupture of the coats of an artery.

An-tē'ri-or. Preceding; before in position; in front.

A'nǔs. The circular opening at the lower extremity of the alimentary canal.

A-or'ta. The great trunk artery of the body.

A-or'tǐc. Pertaining to the aorta.

Ap'er-tūre. An opening; a passage.

A'pěx, pl. Lat. Ap'i-cēs. The tip or summit.

Ap'o-plěx-y. A disease resulting from cerebral hemorrhage, affusion, or from the plugging of a cerebral vessel.

Ap-pā-rā'tus. A complete set of instruments used in performing an operation or experiment.

Ap-pěnd'age". Something attached or annexed.

Ap-pěn-dǐ-cī'tǐs. Inflammation of the vermiform appendix.

A-răch'noid. Membranes, by their extreme thinness, resembling spider-webs.

A-rē'o-lar Tis'sue. Connective or cellular tissue.

Ar'sen-ic (As). A lustrous, crystalline non-metal; in small doses, a general tonic; in large doses, a poison.

Ar-sen-ǐ-oǔs. Pertaining to arsenic.

Ar-sen'ǐ-oǔs ac'id (AsO3). A hard, brittle substance, white oxide of arsenic.

Ar-tē'r'ǐ-ōles. Small arteries.

Ar-ter'i-ō — ve'noǔs. Relating to arteries and veins.

Ar'ter-ī'tǐs. Inflammation of an artery or arteries.

Ar'ter-y. One of the vessels or tubes which conveys the blood from the heart to all parts of the body.

As-ci'tēs. A collection of serous fluid in the abdomen.

As-phyx'ī-āte. To suffocate.

As'pǐr-ā-tor. An instrument for the evacuation of blood or water.

Asth'ma. A disease of respiration.

Ath-er-ō'ma. Fatty degeneration of the walls of the arteries.

Ath-er-ŏ'nia-tous. Pertaining to atheroma.

At-mos-phĕr'ic. Pertaining to the atmosphere.

At'om. The smallest division of matter.

Au'ri-cle. One of the two upper chambers of the heart.

Au-rĭ'cū-lō-vĕn-trĭ'cū-lar Op'ĕn-ĭng. The opening between the auricles and ventricles of the heart.

Au-tŏp'sy. The post-mortem examination of a body.

Ax-ĭl'la. The armpit.

Ax-ĭl'la-ry. Belonging to the axilla or armpit.

Az'y-gos Vein. A vein connecting the superior and inferior venae cavae.

B

Ba-cĭl'lŭs, pl. bacilli. The most important class pathogenically of bacteria.

Ba-cĭl'lŭs In-flu-en'za. A germ believed to cause la grippe.

Ba-cĭl'lŭs Tu-ber-cu-lo'sis. The germ of tuberculosis, or consumption.

Ba-cĭl'lŭs Ty-pho'sus. The germ of typhoid fever.

Ba-cĭl'lŭs of Koch. Germ of Asiatic cholera.

Băc-te'rĭ-a. Microscopic unicellular vegetable organisms found in decaying animal and vegetable matter.

Băc-te'ri-um. An individual of the order of bacteria.

Bas'ĭ-lar. Pertaining to the base, usually of the skull.

Bas'ĭ-lar Ar'ter-y. The artery extending along the border of the Pons Varolii and forming part of the circle of Willis.

Ba-sĭl-ĭc. Vein of the arm used by embalmers in removing blood.

Bī'cĕps. Having two heads.

Bī-chlo'ride. A compound consisting of two atoms of chlorine and one or more atoms of another element.

Bī-cip'ĭ-tal. Relating to biceps muscle.

Bī-cŭs'pĭd. Having two points or cusps.

Bī-fur-cā'tion. Division into two parts.

Bīle. An animal fluid secreted by the liver.

Bī-sĕct'. To divide into two equal parts.

Blăd'der. The reservoir of the urine.

Bor-ac'ic Ac'id (BO_3). The only oxide of boron, antiseptic and crystalline. The most useful salt is borax.

Brăch-ĭ-al. Belonging to the arm, as the brachial artery.

Brāin. The organ of thought, the center of the nervous system.

Bright's Disease. A kidney disease.

Brŏn'chus, pl. brŏn'chī. One of the two subdivisions of the trachea.

Brŏn'chĭ-al. Belonging to the bronchi, as the bronchial tubes.

Bu-bŏn'ĭc. Pertaining to bubo, an inflamed swelling or abscess in glandular parts of the body.

Bŭlb'oŭs. Having bulbs; protuberant.

C

Cad-ă'ver. A dead human body.

Cae'cŭm. Beginning of large intestine.

Cal-car'ĕ-oŭs. Consisting of lime or chalk.

  Căl'cĭ-fĭ-cā'tion. The process of change into a bony substance.

Căl'cĭ'ŭm (Ca). A silver-white metal, the basis of lime.

Ca-năl'. A tubular passage.

Căn'cer. A malignant ttmior.

Căp'ĭl-lar-y, from *capillus,* hair. The minute blood vessels connecting arteries and veins.

Căp'sūle. A small membranous sac investing an organ.

Car-bŏl'ic Ac'id. A crystalline disinfectant.

Car'bon (C). A non-metallic element, abundant in nature.

Car'bon-di-ŏx'ĭde (CO2). A colorless gas, the product of combustion.

Car-bon-ĭ-zā'tion. Conversion into carbon, charging with carbon, or combination with carbon chemically.

Car'di-ăc. Belonging to, or connected with, the heart.

Ca-rŏt'ĭd. Term applied to the two principal arteries of the neck

Car'pŭs. The wrist, composed of eight bones, arranged in two rows.

Car'tĭ-lăge. A smooth, solid and elastic tissue, softer than a bone; gristle.

Car-tĭ-lăg'ĭ-noŭs. Composed of cartilage; gristly.

Căt'a-lĕp-sy. A spasmodic disease, marked by suspension of consciousness and rigidity of the muscles.

Ca-tarrh'. Inflammation of the mucous membrane, especially in the respiratory tract.

Căth'ĕ-ter. An instrument for drawing urine.

Cau-dā'tŭs. One of the lobes of the liver.

Caust'ic. Destructive to organic tissue.

Caust'ic Pot'ash (KO, HO). A white, strongly alkaline solid, potassium hydride.

Cau'ter-ize. To sear or burn with a corrosive substance.

Căv'er-noŭs. Full of caverns; hollow.

Căv'ĭ-ty. A hollow place.

Cell. A closed cavity or sac, the ultimate element in organic structures.

Cell'u-lar. Consisting of, or containing cells.

Ceph-ăl'ĭc. Relating to the head.

Cĕr'-ĕ-brăl or cĕr-ē'bral. Relating to the brain.

Cĕr'ĕ-brō-spī'nal Căv'ĭ-ty. Cavity of brain and spinal cord.

Cĕr'ĕ-brŭm or cĕ-rē'brŭm. The larger and anterior portion of the brain.

Cĕr-ĕ-bĕl'lŭm. Posterior portion of brain.

Cer'vĭ-cal. Pertaining to the neck.

Cĕs-sā'tion. The act of ceasing.

Chām'ber. A cavity.

Chĕm'ĭs-try. The science which investigates the elements of which bodies are composed, their laws of combination and reaction.

Chlor'īde. A compound of chlorine and some other substance.

Chlor'īne (CI). A greenish-yellow, energetic gas.

Chlor-in-ā'ted. Combined, treated or saturated with chlorine.

Chlor'o-phyll. The coloring matter of the green parts of plants.

Chŏl'e-ra. A malignant disease, attended by vomiting and purging.

Chrō'mic Ac'ĭd (Cr_2O_3). An acid of the metal chromium, forming salts of a red or a yellow color.

Chrō-mo'ge-nēs. Supposed vegetable coloring matter acted upon by acids and alkalis to form red, yellow or green tints.

Chrō-mo-gĕn'ĭc. Relating to chromogenes.

Chron'ic. Of long duration.

Chyle. A milky fluid formed in the process of digestion.

Circle of Wil'lis. Anastomosis of the branches of the internal carotid and vertebral arteries at the base of the brain.

Circ-ū-lā'tion. Moving in a circle, as of the blood.

Cir'cū-lā-to-ry. Circulating, or going around.

Cir'cŭm-flĕx. Curved circularly; applied to arteries of the hip, thigh, etc.

Clăv'ĭ-cle. The collar-bone.

Co-ăg'u-lāte. To curdle; to clot.

Cŏc'cyx. A small bone at the end of the sacrum.

Coe'lĭ-ăc Ax'ĭs. A short trunk artery arising from the aorta just below the diaphragm, dividing into the hepatic, gastric and splenic arteries.

Cŏl-lăpse'. To fall together; shrink up.

Cŏl-lăt'er-al Cir-cu-la'tion. Circulation established through indirect or subordinate branches.

Cō'lon. The part of the large intestine connecting caecum and rectum.

Com-mūn'ĭ-ca-ble. Capable of being communicated; as applied to disease, contagious or infectious.

Cŏm-plĕx'us. A muscle in the back of the neck.

Cŏn-cŭs'sion. The shock of agitation of an organ through a fall or blow, as a concussion of the brain.

Cŏn'dyle. A bony process, round in one direction.

Cŏn'dy-loid. Shaped like or pertaining to a condyle.

Cŏn-gĕs'tion. An unnatural accumulation of blood in any part, as congestion of the limgs.

Cŏn'ĭc-al. Having the form of, or resembling a cone.

Cŏn-stĭt'ū-ent. That which constitutes or composes.

Cŏn-strict'ed. Drawn together; contracted.

Cŏn-strict'or. A muscle which contracts.

Cŏn-tā'gion. The transmission of disease, either directly or indirectly, from one person to another.

Cŏn-tā'gioŭs. Communicable by contact.

Cŏn-trăc'tion. The act of drawing together or shrinking.

Cŏn-verge'. To tend to one point.

Cŏn'vĕx. Regularly protuberant or bulging. Opposed to concave.

Cŏn-vŭl'sions. The manifestation of nervous disorder, commonly called fits.

Cŏn-vō-lu'tĕd. Folding or turning back upon itself.

Cŏn'vo-lū'tion. An irregular, tortuous folding of an organ or part.

Cŏr'ă-coid. Resembling a crow's beak.

Cŏr'ō-nā-ry. Encircling.

Corpse. A dead human body.

Corpu-lĕnce. Excessive fatness.

Cor'pus Căl-lō'sum. The great band of commisural fibres uniting the cerebral hemispheres.

Cor-pŭs'cle. A protoplasmic animal cell. Of two kinds, red and white, in the blood.

Cŏr-rō'sĭve. Having the power of consuming away by degrees, as acids do metals.

Cōs-mĕt'ic. A chemical used to. improve the appearance of the skin.

Cŏs'tal. Pertaining to the ribs, as costal cartilages.

Crā'nĭ-ŭm. The bony or cartilaginous case containing the brain.

Crest. The surmounting part of an organ or process.

Cru'ral. Pertaining to the thigh or leg.

Cŭl'ture. A name applied in culture experiments on micro-organisms to the act, the medium used, or the product of the process.

Cu-tā'nĕ-ous. Belonging to the skin or cutis.

Cu'tĭ-cle. Outer skin or epidermis.

Cū'tĭs Ve'ră. True skin.

Cyst. A membranous sac without opening, containing liquid.

Cys'tĭc. Relating to a cyst.

D

Dē-com-pōse'. Resolve into original elements; to decay.

De-gĕn'er-āte. To change from a higher to a lower condition.

De-gĕn'er-ā'tion. Change of tissue from a higher to a lower form,

Dē-jĕc'ta. Faecal matter dejected from the bowels.

Dĕ'mŏn-strāte. To do practical work; to exhibit the parts of a subject.

Dĕnse. Compact; closely united.

Dē-ō'dor-ant. A chemical which destroys odors.

Der'ma. True skin.

Dĕs'ĭc-cāte. To become dry.

Dĕs-ĭc'cant. A substance causing dessication.

Dĕs-ĭc-cā'tion. The process of the removal of moisture from organic tissues.

Dĕt'ri-mSnt. Injury.

Dē-tri'tŭs. Waste matter.

Dī'a-phrăgm. The muscular wall between thorax and abdomen.

Dĭf-fūse'. To pour out or spread, as a liquid.

Dĭf-fū'sion. A spreading or dissemination.

Dĭ-gest'. To prepare for conversion into blood.

Dĭg'ĭ-tal. Pertaining to the fingers.

Dī-lāte'. To expand; opposed to contract.

Dī-ŏx'ide. An oxide containing one equivalent of oxygen to two of a metal.

Dĭph-the'rĭ-a. An infectious disease of the mucous membrane of the air passages.

Dĭph-thĕ-rĭt'ĭc. Pertaining to diphtheria.

Dĭsc. A flat circular plate.

Dis'ĭn-fĕct. To cleanse by the destruction of infectious germs,

Dĭs-ĭn'tĕ-grate. To separate into parts,

Dĭs-sĕct'. To cut for the purpose of scientific examination.

Dĭs-sŏlve'. To separate the parts of a solid body, and cause them to unite with a liquid.

Dĭs'tal. Remote from the place of attachment or the median line.

Dor'sal. Pertaining to the back.

Dor-sal'ĭs Pĕd'ĭs. An artery which is a continuation of the anterior tibial.

Drŏp'sy. A disease attended by accumulation of serous fluid in the cavities or tissues of the body.

Dŭct. A canal for conveying fluid.

Dŭct'ŭs Ar-ter-ĭ-ō'sŭs. A continuation in the foetus of the pulmonary artery.

Dū-ō-dē'nŭm. The first division of the small intestine.

Dū'ra Ma'ter. The outer membrane of the brain.

Dys'ĕn-ter-y. An infectious disease, marked by inflammation of the solitary glands and follicles of the large intestine, together with bloody evacuations.

E

E-clămp'sĭ-a. Convulsions coming on in a woman prior to or during labor.

Ef-fer-vĕs'cence. Bubbling in a liquid, due to escape of gas.

Ef-fēte'. Worn out with age; exhausted.

Em-balm', To preserve from decay.

Em'bo-lĭsm. The obstruction of a vessel by a clot of coagulated blood.

Em'bō-lus. A clot of blood brought by the blood current from a distant artery, and forming an obstruction at its place of lodgment.

Em'bry-ō. The child in the womb before it becomes a foetus;

En-dar-ter-i'tis. Inflammation of the arteries.

En'sĭ-form. Sword-shaped.

En-tĕr'ĭc. Relating to the intestines.

En-te-rī'tĭs. Inflammation of the intestines.

Ep-ĭ-dĕm'ĭc. A prevalent disease.

Ep-ĭ-găs'trĭc. Pertaining to, the superior part of the abdomen; as the epigastric region.

Ep-ĭ-glŏt'tĭs. A cartilage which covers the aperture of the windpipe.

Ep-ĭ-thē'li-al. Pertaining to the cuticle which covers parts deprived of true skin.

Er-y-sĭp'e-las. A disease characterized by inflammation of the skin, swelling, pain and fever.

Eth'moid. Resembling a sieve. Name applied to a bone at the base of the skull.

Eū-stā'chĭ-an Tube. The canal from tympanum to throat or pharytix.

Eū-stā'chĭ-an Valve. A semi-lunar valve, separating the right auricle from the inferior vena cava.

E-vĭs-cer-ā'tion. Removal of the viscera in autopsy.

Ex-crē'ta. The natural discharges of the body, especially of the bowels.

Ex-crēte'. To throw off, as by natural passages.

Ex-cre'tions. The same as excreta.

Ex'cre-to-ry. Having the power of excretion.

Ex-o-spor'ĭ-ŭm. The outer coat of a spore.

Ex-těn'sor. The muscle that extends a limb; opposed to flexor.

Ex-trăv-a-sā'tion. Forcing or being forced out of the proper vessels or ducts.

Ex-trěm'i-ties. Parts remote from median line.

Ex-ū-dā'tion. The oozing of the serum of the blood through the walls of the vessels.

F

Fā'cial. Belonging to the face.

Fa-cul'tā-tive. That form or species of bacteria which may exist either in the living or dead body.

Fae'cal. Pertaining to the faeces.

Fae'cēs. The excretions of the bowels; dejecta.

Făs'ci-a. The layer of tissue immediately beneath the skin.

Fěm'o-ral. Belonging or relating to the thigh, as femoral artery

Fē'mur. The thigh bone.

Fer-měn-tā'tion. Decomposition of an organic substance produced by a ferment.

Fī'bre. A lustrous, slender, thread-like tissue.

Fī'brĭl. A very small fibre.

Fī'brĭne. A white, tough, fibrous substance, the coagulum of the blood.

Fī'brĭ-noŭs. Having fibrin.

Fī'broŭs. Containing or consisting of fibres.

Fĭb'ū-la. The small, outer bone of the leg.

Fĭs'sion. Reproduction by division.

Fĭs'sūre. A groove or depression.

Flesh. The soft tissues of the body, especially the muscles.

Flěx'or. A muscle which bends a limb or part.

Flěx'or Car'pi Ra-di-a'lis. A muscle on the radial side of the forearm.

Flex'or Car'pi Ul-nar'is. A muscle on the thumb side of the forearm.

Flěx-ure. A bending or curving.

Flōat'er. A term applied to a floating dead body.

Flu'orine (Fl). A gaseous element having a powerful affinity for hydrogen.

Foe'tal. Pertaining to the foetus.

Foe'tŭs. The product of conception from the fourth month to the end of pregnancy.

Fŏ-rā'měn. A small opening. An opening in the bones through which nerves or blood-vessels pass.

Fo-rā'men Cae'cŭm. The blind passage at the root of the spine of the frontal bone.

Fo-rā'men Mag'num. An opening in the occipital bone communicating with the spinal canal.

Fōre'arm. That part of the arm below the elbow.

For'ma-lin. A proprietary name for formaldehyde.

For-măl'dě-hyde. A colorless volatile fluid (H_2CO); a powerful disinfectant.

For'mĭc Ac'ĭd. A liquid contained in a fluid emitted by red ants. Now obtained by artificial distillation.

Fŏs'sa. A depression, furrow or sinus.

Frŏnt'al. Relating to the forehead.

Fūm-ĭ-gā'tion. Disinfection by exposure to fumes of a vaporized disinfectant.

Fŭnc'tion. The normal or special action of a tissue or part.

G

Gall. A bitter, yellowish-green fluid secreted by the liver; the bile.

Găn'grēne. The first stage of mortification; the death of a part.

Găs. Any substance normally in aeriform condition.

Găs'eous. In the form of, or containing, gas.

Găs'tric. Belonging to the stomach.

Gě-lăt'ĭ-noŭs. Having the nature of gelatine or jelly.

Gěn'er-āt-ing. Producing.

Gěn'er-ā-tĭve. Having the power of generation.

Germ. The ovum or spore which, by fecundation, develops into an organism like that from which it is derived.

Germ-ĭ-cīdes'. Disinfectants destructive to bacteria or germs.

Germ-ĭ-cī'dal. Pertaining to germicides; destructive to germs.

Gěs-tā'tion. The bearing of the young in the womb; pregnancy.

Glănd. An organ excretive and secretive in function.

Gland'ers. A contagious and fatal disease of the mucous membrane.

Glăn'du-lar. Pertaining to glands.

Glŏb'ūle. A small globe-shaped particle of matter.

Glŏb'ū-lin. The principal constituent of blood globules; closely allied to albumen.

Grăph-īte. A soft, black, lustrous substance. Pure graphite is carbon.

Grăv-ĭ-tā'tion. The tendency of every particle of matter towards every other particle.

Groin. The depression between the abdomen and thigh.

Gŭl'lĕt. See oesophagus.

H

Hae'mō-glō-bĭn. The coloring matter of the red corpuscles of the blood; it serves to convey oxygen to the tissues in circulation.
Hĕm'ĭ-spheres. The halves of the cerebrum.
Hĕm'or-rhoids. Tubercles around or within the anus; piles.
Hĕ-păt'ĭc. Belonging or relating to the liver.
Hī'lŭm. That part of a gland or similar organ where the bloodvessels enter.
Hun'ter's Can-al'. A triangular space between three muscles of the leg.
Hū'mēr-ŭs. The bone of the upper arm.
Hy'drō-cēle. Dropsy of the testicle.
Hy-drō-cĕph'a-lŭs. Dropsy of the brain.
Hy-drō-chlor'ĭc Ac'ĭd (HCl). An acid of chlorine much used in chemical laboratories.
Hy'drō-gĕn (H). A colorless, odorless, gaseous element, the lightest known substance.
Hy'gĭ-ēne. The science of health.
Hy'oid. A tiny, arch-shaped bone at the root of the tongue.
Hy-pō-chŏn'drĭ-ăc. One who is morbidly melancholy.
Hy-pō-der'mĭc. Pertaining to the parts beneath the skin.
Hy-pō-găs'trĭc. Pertaining to lower part of abdomen.
Hys-te'rĭ-a. A functional disturbance of the nervous system
Hys-tĕr'ĭc-al. Affected with, or suffering from hysteria.

I

Il'ĕ-ăc. Relating to the ileum.
Il'ĕ-ŏ-cae'căl. Relating to both ileum and caecum.
Il'ĕ-ŭm. The last division of the small intestine.
Il'ĭ-ăc. Pertaining to the ilium.
Il'ĭ-ŭm. Upper part of os innominatum.
Im-mūne'. Capable of resisting contagion or infection.
Im-prĕg'nāte. To cause to conceive.
In-cī'sion, A cut.
In-fĕct'. To taint with disease.
In-fĕc'tious. Easily communicated; contagious.
In-fer'ĭ-ŏr. Lower in position or in importance.
In-flam-mā'tion. A morbid condition attended by heat, redness, pain or swelling.
In-flu-ĕn'za. . An epidemic affection of the mucous membrane of the respiratory tract, accompanied by fever.
In-fu-so'rĭ-a. Microscopic, unicellular, vegetable organisms found in infusions of decaying animal and vegetable matter.

In'guĭn-al. Pertaining to the groin.

In-nŏc'u-oŭs. Harmless.

In-ŏc'u-lāte. To communicate a disease by injection of infectious matter in the flesh.

In-or-găn'ĭc. Not produced by vital action.

In-ŏs'cu-lāte. To cause to unite or grow together.

In-sol-ā'tion. Sunstroke.

In-spĭ-rā'tion. The drawing in of the breath.

In-tĕg'u-mĕnt. A covering; the skin.

In-ter-cŏs'tal. Between the ribs.

In-ter-mĭt'tent. Occurring at intervals.

Inter-ŏs'sĕ-oŭs. Between the bones.

In'ter-spāce. Intervening space.

In-tĕs'tĭ-nal. Pertaining to the intestines.

In-tĕs'tĭnes. The bowels.

In-vŏl'ŭn-ta-ry. Not dependent upon the will.

I-ŏd'o-form (CHI3). An antiseptic and anaesthetic compound of iodine used as a local application for wounds and sores.

Is'chĭ-ŭm. The hip bone.

J

Jaun'dĭce. A disease arising from disorder of the liver, characterized by yellow discoloration of the skin.

Jĕ-jŭn'ŭm. The second division of the small intestine.

Jū'gu-lar. Belonging to the throat or neck.

Junc'tion. Union; joint.

K

Kĭd'nĕys. The two large glandular organs of the lumbar region which secrete urine.

Kre'sol (C7H8O). An aromatic alcohol of the benzene group.

L

Lăc'er-āt-ĕd. Torn asunder.

Lăch'rym-al. Pertaining to, or secreting tears.

Lăc'tĕ-als. The vessels which convey chyle.

Lăc'tĭc. An acid, derived chiefly from sour milk.

Lăr'ynx. The organ of voice.

Lăt'er-al. Pertaining to the sides.

Lĕp'ro-sy. A chronic and malignant disease, prevalent in the Old World, and characterized by tubercular lesions of the skin.

Lē'sion. A rupture or tearing of the flesh; a wound.

Lĭg'a-mĕnt. A tough band of fibrous tissue uniting bones, or holding organs in position.

Lĭg'a-tūre. A thread for tying blood-vessels to prevent hemorrhage.

Lĭn'ĕ-ar. Pertaining to a line or lines.

Lĭn'gual. Of, or pertaining to the tongue.

Lĭ'quĕ-fy. To make or to become liquid.

Lĭv'er. The largest glandular organ of the body, whose principal function is to secrete bile.

Löbe. A rounded and projecting part of an organ.

Lŏb'u-lar. Like a lobule.

Lŏb'ule. A small lobe; lobulus.

Lŏb'u-lŭs Qua-dra'tus. The square lobe under the right lobe of the liver.

Lŏb'u-lŭs Spi-gel'ĭ-i. The lobule projecting from the back part of the under surface of the liver.

Lŏn'gĭ-tud'ĭn-al. Running lengthwise.

Lŏn'gus. Long.

Lŭm'bar. Pertaining to the loins.

Lymph. A whitish fluid of the lymphatic vessels.

Lym-phăt'ĭcs. Fine absorbent tubes pervading the body.

Ly'sol. Phenol from cresols by action of nascent soap; an excellent disinfectant in from 1 to 3 per cent solutions.

M

Măg-nē'sĭ-a (MgO). The oxide of magnesium, a white powder used in medicine.

Măg-nē'sĭ-ŭm (Mg). One of the more abundant elements which forms an important part of the earth's crust.

Mag-nē'si-um Sŭl'phāte (MgSO4, 7H2O). The most important salt of magnesium.

Mā'lar. Pertaining to the cheek or to the malar bone.

Ma-lā'ri-a. Bad or infected air.

Ma-lār'ĭ-al Fē'ver. Fever caused by malaria.

Ma-lĭg'nant. Threatening a fatal issue; virulent.

Măl-lĕ-o'lŭs. One of the projections of the bones of the leg at the ankle joint.

Măs'toid. Shaped like the nipple or breast.

Măx-ĭl'la. A jaw bone.

Măx'ĭl-lăry. Pertaining to the jaw; properly, restricted to the upper jaw.

Mēas'les. An acute, infectious disease, characterized by fever, catarrh and eruption,

Mē'dĭ-an. Central in position.

Mĕ-dĭ-ăs'tĭn-al. Pertaining to the mediastinum.

Mĕ-dĭ-ăs-tī'nŭm. Septum formed by the union of the pleurae.

Mĕ-dŭl'la. Marrow.

Me-dŭl'a Ob'lŏn-gā'ta. The upper portion of the spinal cord.

Mĕm'brāne. A thin tissue serving to cover some part of the body or to absorb and secrete fluids.

Mĕm-brā'ne-oŭs / Mĕm-brā-noŭs. Consisting of, or relating to membrane.

159

Mer'cu-ry (Hg). A silver-white metal; quicksilver.

Měs'ĕn-tĕr'ĭc. Pertaining to the mesentery.

Měs'ĕn-tĕr-y. A fold of peritoneum, connecting intestine with abdominal wall.

Mět-a-car'pal. Belonging to that part of the hand between wrist and fingers.

Mět-a-mor'phō-sĭs. Change of form or structure.

Mět-a-tar'sal. Belonging to that part of the foot between ankle and toes.

Mī'crōbe. The general name for micro-organisms.

Mī-crō-cŏc'cŭs (kŏk'kŭs), pl. micrococci (sī). A species of bacteria shaped like dumb-bells, or in the form of oval cells, forming chains.

Mī'crō-or'gan-ism. A minute organism.

Mĭn'er-al. Any chemical combination containing an organic base found in the earth.

Mĭt'ĭ-gā-ted. Allayed, eased.

Mī'tral. Shaped like a mitre; having two points.

Mŏl'ĕ-cūle. The smallest particle of matter that can exist uncombined.

Mor'bĭd. Diseased; in an abnormal state.

Morgue. Place where unknown dead are kept for recognition.

Mor'phine. An alkaloid of opium.

Mor'tal. Subject to death.

Mor-tĭf-ĭ-cā'tion. Death of one part of a living body; gangrene.

Mouth. An opening. The entrance to the alimentary canal.

Mū'coŭs. Pertaining to or resembling mucus.

Mū'cŭs. A viscid fluid secreted by the mucous membrane, which it serves to keep moist.

Mū-rĭ-ăt'ĭc. Pertaining to, or obtained from sea salt.

Mŭs'cles. Organs of motion; the lean meat of the body.

Mŭs'cu-lar. Pertaining to, or consisting of, muscle; strong.

My-ō'sĭn. The clot formed in the coagulation of muscle plasma.

Myrrh (mer). A transparent juice which exudes from the bark of an Arabian shrub.

N

Nar-cŏt'ĭc. A medicine producing sleep.

Nā'sal. Pertaining to the nose.

Nā'tron (NaO_6CO_2, $10H_2O$). The native carbonate of soda.

Nā'vel. A mark in the centre of the abdomen.

Nerve. A bundle of fibres which establish communication between the nerve centres and other parts of the body.

Nerv'oŭs. Pertaining to the nerves.

Nī'trate. A salt of nitric acid.

Nī'tric Ac'id (HNO_3). A powerful, corrosive acid.

Nī'tre. Saltpetre (KO, NO_5).

Nī'tro-gĕn. A gaseous element, forming nearly four-fifths of the atmosphere.

Nor'mal. According to rule; regular.

Nū'cle-ā-ted. Gathered about a nucleus or centre.

Nū'cle-ŭs. A central mass or point about which matter is gathered.

Nū'trĭ-ent. Nourishing; that which nourishes.

Nū'trĭ-mĕnt. That which promotes growth and repairs waste.

Nū-trĭ'tion. That which nourishes; the process of growth and repair.

O

Ob-strŭc'tion. The act of stopping or closing up. An obstacle; a hindrance.

Oc-cĭp'i-tal. Pertaining to the back part of the head.

Oe-dē'ma. Dropsy of a part.

Oe-sŏ-phăg'ĕ-al. Pertaining to the oesophagus.

Oe-sŏph'a-gŭs. The tube through which food passes from mouth to stomach.

O-mĕn'tum. A fold of peritoneum, covering the bowels and attached to the stomach.

Opāque (o-pak'). Not transparent; dark.

Op-er-ā'tion. An act performed with the hand or with instruments on the body.

Or-bĭc'u-lar. (Circular.

Or-bic-u-lā'ris. A circular muscle.

Or'gan. A part of the body of special function.

Or-găn'ĭc. Pertaining to an organ or its functions; consisting of organs.

Or'gan-ĭsm. A being endowed with organs.

Or'ĭ-fĭce (or'ĭ-fĭs). An opening.

Os-mō'sĭs. The tendency of fluids to pass through animal membranes.

Os'sa In-nŏm'ĭn-a'ta. The hip bones.

Os'sĕ-oŭs. Composed of bone; bony.

Os-sĭ-fĭ-cā'tion. The change into a bony substance.

O-vār'ĭ-an. Of or relating to the ovary.

O'var-y. The sexual glands of the female containing the ova.

Ox-ăl'ĭc Ac'id (C (OH)$_3$ — C (OH)$_3$). A caustic, dibasic acid of the urine.

Ox'īde. A compound of oxygen with a metal or metalloid.

Ox'y-gen. A tasteless, odorless, colorless element, forming about twenty-two per cent of the atmosphere.

Ox'y-gĕn-at'ĕd. Combined with oxygen.

P

Păb'u-lŭm. Food.

Palm. The inner part of the hand from wrist to fingers.

Păl'mar. Of or relating to the palm.

Păn'crĕ-ăs. A whitish, irregular shaped gland, situated deep in the abdomen, behind the stomach.

Păn-crĕ-ăt'ĭc. Pertaining to the pancreas.

Pa-răl'y-sĭs. Complete or partial loss of voluntary motion.

Păr'ă-sīte. An animal or plant which preys upon other living bodies.

Pa-rī'ĕt-al. Pertaining to the bones which form the sides of the skull.

Pa-rŏt'ĭd. The salivary nearest to the ear. Pertaining to the parotid.

Par'ŏx-ysm. The attack of an intermittent disease. A fit.

Păs'sage. Way or course.

Pa-tĕl'la. The knee-pan.

Path-o-gĕn'ĭc. Productive of diseases.

Pa-thŏlo-gy. The science of diseases.

Pĕc'to-ral. Pertaining to the breast.

Pē'dēs. Plural of *pes,* a foot.

Pĕl'vĭc. Pertaining to the pelvis.

Pĕl'vĭs. The basin formed by the innominate bones and the sacrum.

Pĕl-lū'cĭd. Clear, but not transparent.

Pĕr-ĭ-car-di'tĭs. Inflammation of the pericardium.

Pĕr-ĭ-car'dĭ-um (per-e-kar'de-um). The membranous sac which encloses the heart.

Pĕ-riph'er-al. External, bounding.

Pĕr-ĭ-stăl'sĭs. A movement peculiar to the intestines; a narrowing from above downward, forcing along the food.

Pĕr-ĭ-stăl'tĭc-al-ly. In the manner of peristalsis.

Per-măn'ga-nate. A salt of permanganic acid ($HMnO_4$).

Pĕr'mĕ-ate. To penetrate or pass through.

Per-ŏx'ĭde. Of two or more compounds of oxygen with the same element, that which contains the largest relative amount of oxygen.

Pĕ-trōs'al. Pertaining to the petrous portion of the temporal bone.

Pē'troŭs. Hard or stony.

Pha-lăn'gēs. The small bones of the fingers and toes.

Phă-ryn'gĕ-al. Belonging to, or connected with, the pharynx.

Phăr'ynx (far'inks). The upper part of the throat.

Phĕ-nŏm'ĕn-ŏn. Something remarkable or unusual.

Phŏs'phor-ŭs. A nearly colorless, combustible, non-metallic element, in physical properties resembling fine wax.

Phrĕn'ĭc (frĕn'ik). Belonging to the diaphragm.

Phys'ĭc-al (fĭz'ik-al). Pertaining to nature; obeying the laws of nature.

Pī'a Mā'ter. The vascular membrane immediately investing the brain.

Pĭg'mĕnt. Coloring matter.

Pī'sĭ-form. Having form and size of a pea.

Pit. An indenture in the flesh. The mark left by a pustule of the small -pox.

Pit of Stomach. The hollow of the stomach. Portion of the abdomen above the waist or belly.

Plă-cĕn'ta. The soft, vascular disc which connects the mother with the child in the womb, and through which the foetus draws nourishment.

Pla-cĕn'tal. Pertaining to the placenta.

Plăn'tar. Pertaining to the sole of the foot.

Plăs'ma. The colorless fluid of the blood.

Plas'ter of Paris. Calcined gypsum or sulphate of lime.

Pleū'ra. The serous membrane which lines the thorax and invests the lungs.

Pleū'rĭ-sy. Inflammation of the pleura.

Pleu-rī'tĭs. Pleurisy.

Plĕx'ŭs. A network of vessels, nerves or fibres.

Pneu'mō-cŏc'cŭs. A germ believed to cause pneumonia.

Pneu-mō'nĭ-a. Inflammation of the lungs.

Pŏck-mark. The mark left by a pustule.

Pŏns Va-rō'lĭ-ī (Lat. *pons,* a bridge). Part of the brain.

Pŏp-lĭ-tē'al. Pertaining to the posterior part of the knee joint.

Pŏp-n-te'ŭs. A muscle in the back and lower part of the thigh.

Port'al. Pertaining to the porta or gateway of the liver; as, the portal vein.

Pŏs-ter'ĭ-or. Behind in position.

Pōst-mor'tem. After death.

Pŏ-tăs'sĭ-ŭm (K). An abundant, silver-white metal, readily oxidized.

Pou'part's Lig'a-mĕnt. A ligament extending from the spine of the ileum to the pubis.

Prĕg'nan-cy. The state of being pregnant.

Prĕg'nant. With child.

Prō'cĕss. A protuberance or projecting part of any surface; usually a bone.

Pro-fŭn'da. A name applied to an artery.

Prō-nāt'or. A muscle which serves to bend the palm of the hand downward; opposed to supinator.

Prō-sĕc'tor. A person who prepares a cadaver for lectures and demonstrations.

Prō'tĕ-ids. Albuminoid compounds.

Prō'tō-plăsm. The mucilaginous, granular matter of cells; the physical basis of life.

Prŏ-tū'ber-ance. A swelling or prominence.

Pū'bes. The anterior part of the pelvis.

Pū'bĭc. Pertaining to the pubes.

Pū'bĭs. Anterior part of one of the hip bones.

Pu-er'per-al. Pertaining to child-birth.

Pŭl'mōn-a-ry. Pertaining to the lungs.

Pŭlse. The beating of the heart or of a blood-vessel, especially of an artery.

Pŭnct'ūre. The act of perforating with a pointed instrument.

Pu'pĭl. The small opening in the center of the iris.

Purging. Cleansing or purifying by the removal of that which is impure or foreign.

Pur'pū-ra. An unhealthy condition of the blood and tissues, evinced by purple spots on the skin.

Pūr'u-lent. Containing pus.

Pŭs. A yellowish, creamy liquid, the product of inflammation.

Pŭst'ūle. An inflamed elevation of the cuticle containing pus.

Pu-trĕ-făc'tion. Decomposition; offensive decay.

Pu-trĕ-făc'tĭve. Pertaining to putrefaction.

Py-ē'mĭ-a. A dangerous disease, caused by poisonous pus in the blood; blood poisoning.

Py-lŏr'ĭc. Pertaining to the pylorus.

Py-lōr'ŭs. The opening in the stomach through which the food passes to the small intestines.

R

Rā'dĭ-al. Pertaining to the radius.

Răd'ĭ-cal. Reaching to the center or foundation. A molecule that preserves its integrity, either as a base or as an acid.

Rā'dĭ-us. The long bone on the thumb side of the forearm.

Răm'ĭ-fy. To divide into branches.

Rĕc'tum. The large intestine from sigmoid flexure to anus.

Rē-gur'gĭ-tāte. To return, or flow back.

Rē-gur'gĭ-tā'tion. A flowing backward or reflex, as of blood in incompetent heart valves, or of food or liquid that has been swallowed.

Rē'nal. Pertaining to the kidneys.

Res'er-voir' (rez'er-vwor') . A place where anything is kept in store.

Rĕs-pĭ-rā'tion. The act of breathing.

Rĕ-spir'ă-to-ry. Pertaining to respiration.

Rē'tĕ Mū-cō'sum. The layer of epidermis lying next to the corium into which the papillae of the skin project.

Rĕt'ĭ-na. The sensitive and innermost coat of the eye, formed by the expansion of the optic nerve.

Rheū'mă-tĭsm. Painful inflammation, acute or chronic, affecting muscles and joints.

Rĭg'or Mor'tĭs. Rigidity of the body after death.

Rōp'y. Stringy; adhesive; viscous.

Rŭp'tūre. Breaking or laceration of the walls or continuity of an organ.

S

Săc. A pouch-like structure.

Sā'crŭm. A bone in the lower part of the back.

Săl'ĭ-cyl'ĭc Ac'ĭd (C_7 H_6 O_3). An aromatic acid of salicin, occurring in various essential oils.

Sa-lī'va. A transparent liquid secreted by the salivary glands.

Salts. Popular name for Epsom salts or magnesium sulphate.

Săn'i-tar-y. Relating to the preservation of health.

Săn-ĭ-tā'tion. The adoption of sanitary measures.

Sa-phē'na. One of the two subcutaneous veins of the lower limb and foot.

Sa-phē'nous. The two principal superficial veins of the lower limbs.

Săp'rō-phyt'ĭc. Pertaining to a saprophyte.

Săp'rō-phyte. A plant that lives on decomposing organic substances.

Scar-la-tī'na. See scarlet fever.

Scar'let Fē'ver. A contagious disease characterized by a scarlet eruption of the skin.

Scarpa's Tri'an-gle. A triangle formed by Poupart's ligaments above, sartorius muscles without, and adductor longus within.

Scrōt'al. Pertaining to the scrotum.

Scrō'tŭm. The sac which contains the testes.

Sĕ-crē'tion. The separation from the blood; collection and discharge of various fluid or semi-fluid substances; a natural function of certain organs.

Sĕm'i-lu'nar. Resembling a half moon in shape.

Sĕp-a-rāt'ĭng Mĕm'brāne. A membranous portion.

Sĕp'ta. Plural of septum.

Sĕp'tĭc. Promoting putrefaction; a substance which promotes putrefaction. ,

Sĕp-tĭ-ce'mi-ă,. Blood poisoning.

Sĕp'tŭm. A membranous partition separating two cavities.

Ser'oŭs. Pertaining to serum; thin; watery.

Ser'ŭm. A fluid of serous cavities.

Sheath (shēth). A thin covering.

Sĭg'moid. Curved like the letter S.

Sĭg'moid Flex'ure. The last curve of the colon.

Sĭl'ĭ-ca. Silicon dioxide, (SiO_2) in its purest form, quartz.

Sĭl'ĭ-cŏn (Si). After oxygen, the most important element of the earth's crust.

Sī'nus. A venous channel into which several vessels empty, especially those of the dura mater.

Skĕl'e-ton. The bony framework of the body.

Skŭll., The bony framework of the cranium and face.

Small'pŏx. A malignant disease, characterized by pustular eruptions.

So'di-ŭm (Na). A yellowish, metallic element, lighter than water.

Sō'di-ŭm Chlo'rĭde (NaCl). Common salt.

So'di-ŭm Sŭl'phāte (Na_2SO_4). Glauber's salts. Salt of sodium of medicinal value.

Sō-lū'tion. The infusion of the molecules of a solid, liquid, or gaseous substance among those of a liquid.

Sŏl'vent, Able to dissolve. A fluid containing a substance in solution.

Spăs'm. The involuntary and abnormal contraction of one or more muscles.

Spăs'mŏd'ic. Relating to a spasm; convulsive.

Spē'ciēs (spē'shēz) . A group of organisms having similar characteristics.

Spē-cĭf'ĭc. Pertaining to a species; definite.

Sper-măt'ĭc. Pertaining to the semen.

Sphăc'ĕ-lŭs. The gangrenous part.

Sphēn'oid / Sphēn-oid'al. Resembling a wedge. The sphenoid bone is at the base of the skull on the median line.

Spīne. The back-bone or spinal column.

Spī'nal. Pertaining to the spine.

Spi-rĭl'lŭm, pl. spi-rĭl'la. A genus of bacteria, spiral in shape.

Spleen. A ductless oval organ just below the diaphragm on the left side.

Splĕn'ĭc. Relating to the spleen.

Spore. A specialized cell capable of developing into a new individual.

Spū'tŭm, pl. spū'ta. Matter expectorated from the mouth.

Stĕr'ĭle. Unfruitful; producing no young.

Stĕr'ĭl-īze. To make sterile. To destroy microbes in.

Stern'al. Pertaining ,to the sternum.

Ster'no-măs'toid. Pertaining to the stemimi and to the mastoid process of the temporal bone.

Ster'nŭm. The flat bone in the median line in the front of the chest.

Stĕth'ō-scōpe. An instrument for testing the condition of the heart and lungs by the sounds within the chest.

Stom'ach (stŭm'ak). The third division of the alimentary canal, of excessive digestive power.

Strĭc'tūre. A morbid contraction.

Strōke. A sudden attack of disease.

Strŭc'tūre. The arrangement of parts.

Sŭb-clā'vĭ-an. Beneath the clavicle, or collar-bone.

Sŭb-cū-tā'nĕ-oŭs. Situated beneath the skin.

Sŭb'lĭm-āte. A product of vaporization and condensation.

Sŭb-scăp'ŭ-lar. Beneath the scapula.

Sŭc'cu-lent. Juicy.

Sŭlph'āte. A salt of sulphuric acid.

Sŭl'phur (S). A non-metallic, crystalline element, yellow in color.

Sŭl'phu-roŭs. Containing sulphur.

Sŭl'phu-roŭs Ac'id (H_2SO_3). An acid of sulphur.

Sū-per-fĭc'ial (Sū'per-fish'al) . Near the surface.

Sū-pēr'ĭ-or. Higher; above in position.

Sū'pĭ-nāt-or Long'us. A muscle that turns the palm of the hand upward.

Sŭp-pū-rā'tion. The formation or discharge of pus.

Sū'pra or sū'per. A prefix signifying above, over or beyond.

Sū-pra-rē'nal. Above the kidneys.

Sū'tūre (sūt'yur). A line formed by the union of two parts; the sutures of the skull are the seams or joints of the bones.

Syn'cō-pĕ. Fainting; apparent cessation of action in heart, lungs, brain, etc.

Sym'phy-sĭs. Union of bones by an immovable joint.

Symp-tō-măt'ĭc. Pertaining to a symptom.

Syph'ĭ-lĭs. An infectious venereal disease.

Syph-ĭ-lĭt'ĭc. Pertaining to syphilis.

Sys'tem. Parts methodically arranged to form a whole, and having a definite function.

Sys-tĕm'ĭc. Belonging to the whole body.

T

Tar'sal. Pertaining to the ankle.

Těm'pōr-al. Pertaining to the temple or temples.

Těn'dĭn-oŭs. Of, or pertaining to, a tendon.

Těn'don. A strong, glistening, fibrous cord, attaching a muscle to a bone.

Těs'tĭ-cle, pl. test'ēs. One of the glands which secrete the seminal fluid in males.

Tět'an-ŭs. Contraction of the muscles, causing rigidity.

Thŏ-răc'ĭc. Relating to the thorax.

Thor'ăx. The trunk from neck to diaphragm; the chest.

Thym'ol ($C_{10}H_{14}O$). A crystalline antiseptic, soluble in alcohol and ether.

Thrŏm-bō'sĭs. The formation of a thrombus.

Thrŏm'bŭs. A clot of blood.

Thyr'oid. Resembling a shield. The thyroid cartilage is often called "Adam's apple."

Tĭb'ĭ-ă. The skin bone larger than the fibula.

Tĭb'ĭ-al. Pertaining to the tibia.

Tĭss'ūe. The texture of organs or parts of organs.

Tor'tū-oŭs. Winding; twisted.

Trā'chĕ-a. The wind-pipe.

Trăn-sū-dā'tion. A passing through; as through pores.

Trăns-verse'. Extending across, or in a crosswise direction.

Tra-pē'zĭ-ŭs. A muscle of the back, whose action is to draw the head backward.

Trĭb'ū-tar-y. Subordinate.

Trī'cĕps. A three-headed muscle of the arm, whose action is to extend the forearm.

Tri-cus'pĭd. Having three cusps or points.

Tri-kre'sol ($C_7H_8O_2$). A colorless, caustic antiseptic.

True Skin. Term often applied to the cutis.

Trŭnk. The body apart from the head and limbs.

Tū'ber-cle. A growth, in the shape of minute rounded masses, apt to spring up in lungs.

Tubercle Bacilli. The bacilli or germs of tuberculosis, rod-shaped, with rounded ends.

Tu-ber'cu-loŭs. Having tubercles; pertaining to tubercles.

Tu-ber-cū-lo'sĭs. A disease caused by tuberculous bacteria; consumption.

Tūb'u-lar. Having the form of a tube or pipe.

Tū'mōr. A morbid swelling or growth.

Tur'bĭn-āt-ĕd. Shaped like an inverted cone.

Ty'phoid. Of or pertaining to typhus.

Typhoid Fever. A continued fever, due to the virus, bacillus typhosis, characterized by intestinal lesions, diarrhoea, prostration, etc.

Ty-phō'sĭs. Referring to bacillus of typhoid fever.

Ty'phŭs. A continuous fever, lasting from two to three weeks, and attended with brain disorder.

U

Ul-cer-ā'tion. The formation of an ulcer.

Ul-na (ul'nah). The distal and larger of the two bones of the forearm.

Ul'nar. Pertaining to the ulna.

Um-bĭl'ĭc-al. Pertaining to the umbilicus or navel.

Umbilical Cord. The cord connecting the placenta of the mother with the navel of the foetus.

Um-bĭl'ĭ-cŭs. The scar at the median line of the abdomen, caused by the detachment of the umbilical cord after birth.

U-rē'ter. One of the two tubes which convey the urine from the kidney to the bladder.

U-rē'thră. The canal by which the urine passes from the bladder.

Ur'in-ar-y. Pertaining to the urine.

Ur'ĭne. The fluid secreted by the kidneys and discharged by the bladder.

U'ter-īne. Pertaining to the uterus or womb.

U'ter-ŭs. A hollow, pear-shaped, muscular organ in the pelvic cavity of the female, between bladder and rectum, in which the foetus is conceived and nourished.

V

Văc'cĭ-nāte. To inoculate with the cow-pox.

Văc-cĭ-nā'tion. The act of vaccinating.

Văc'ū-ŭm. Space empty; devoid of air or any material substance.

Va-gī'na. Canal from vulval opening to neck of womb.

Vălve. A membranous partition which opens to allow passage of fluid and closes to prevent its regurgitation.

Văr'ĭ-cōse. Swollen or enlarged.

Vā'ri-loid. A modified form of small-pox.

Văs'cu-lar. Consisting of, or containing vessels.

Vein (vān). A vessel which returns the blood from capillaries to heart.

Vē'na. A vein.

Vē'nae The-bē'sĭ-ī. The small veins which assist in returning the blood from the walls of the heart to the right auricle.

Vĕ-ner'ĕ-al. Arising from sexual intercourse.

Vē-noŭs. Of or pertaining to veins.

Vĕn'trĭ-cle. A cavity; especially the lower cavities of the heart.

Vĕn-trĭc'ū-lar. Of or pertaining to a ventricle.

Ver'mĭ-form. Shaped like a worm.

Vermiform appendix. A blind pouch projecting from the caecum.

Ver'tĕ-bra, pl. vertebrae. One oi the bones of the spinal column.

Ver'tĕ-bral. Of or pertaining to the vertebrae.

Ver'tĕx. The highest point.

Vĕs'sel. A tube through which fluids of the body, especially the blood, circulate.

Vĭr'u-lent. Extremely poisonous.

Vīr'ŭs. Poisonous matter.

Vĭs'cer-a, pl. of viscus. Organs of the great cavities.

Vis'cer-al. Pertaining to the viscera.

Vĭs'cĭd. Sticky.

Vī'tăl. Pertaining to life.

Vŏl'ŭn-tar-y. Regulated by the will.

Vō'mer. A slender, thin bone separating the nostrils.

W

Wind'pipe. The trachea.

Womb (wōōm). The uterus where the child is conceived and nourished.

Y

Yellow Fever. A malignant disease of warm climates.

Z

Zyme (zīm). A ferment.

www.ingramcontent.com/pod-product-compliance
Lightning Source LLC
Chambersburg PA
CBHW032000190326
41520CB00007B/309